PHARMACOLOGY AND DRUG ADMINISTRATION

for Imaging Technologists

PHARMACOLOGY AND DRUG ADMINISTRATION
for Imaging Technologists

STEVEN C. JENSEN, Ph.D., R.T. (R.)

Director of Radiologic Sciences,
College of Applied Sciences and Arts,
Health Care Professions,
Southern Illinois University,
Carbondale, Illinois

MICHAEL P. PEPPERS, Pharm.D., R.Ph.

Regional Pharmacy Manager,
Apria Health Care, Inc.,
St. Louis, Missouri

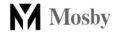 Mosby

St. Louis Baltimore Boston Carlsbad Chicago Minneapolis New York Philadelphia Portland
London Milan Sydney Tokyo Toronto

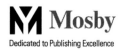
Mosby
Dedicated to Publishing Excellence

A Times Mirror
Company

Publisher: Don Ladig
Senior Editor: Jeanne Rowland
Developmental Editor: Carole Glauser
Project Manager: Mark Spann
Production Editor: Steve Hetager
Book Design Manager: Gail Morey Hudson
Cover Design: Teresa Breckwoldt
Manufacturing Supervisor: Debbie LaRocca

Printed in the United States of America
Composition by Top Graphics
Printing/binding by R.R. Donnelley & Sons Company

Mosby, Inc.
11830 Westline Industrial Drive
St. Louis, Missouri 64146

www.mosby.com

International Standard Book Number 0-8151-4894-1

98 99 00 01 02 / 9 8 7 6 5 4 3 2 1

Reviewers

CHARLEEN GOMBERT, B.R., R.T.(T.), R.N.
Program Director,
Radiation Therapy Technology Program,
Community College of Allegheny County,
Pittsburgh, Pennsylvania

GINGER S. GRIFFIN, R.T.(R.), F.A.S.R.T.
Program Director,
School of Radiologic Technology,
Baptist Medical Center,
Jacksonville, Florida

DIANE H. GRONEFELD, M.Ed., R.T.(R.)
Associate Professor,
Radiologic Technology Program,
Northern Kentucky University,
Highland Heights, Kentucky

DAVID S. HALL, M.S., R.T.(R.)
Associate Professor,
Radiologic Sciences Program,
Broward Community College,
Davie, Florida

SHERI L. HOSTERMAN, A.S., R.T.(R.)(C.V.)
Clinical Instructor,
School of Radiologic Technology,
Holy Spirit Hospital,
Camp Hill, Pennsylvania

DAVID G. HRINO, R.T.(R.)(C.T.)
Continuing Education Consultant,
CT Technologist,
Gnaden Huetten Memorial Hospital,
Lehighton, Pennsylvania

MICHAEL A. KLEINHOFFER, B.S., R.T.(R.)
Clinical Research Associate,
Novartis Pharmaceuticals Corporation,
Highland, Illinois

JOSEPHINE M. LATINI, M.S., R.T.(R.)
Assistant Manager of Radiology,
Department of Radiology,
Lock Haven Hospital,
Lock Haven, Pennsylvania

ART MEYERS, Ed.D., R.T.(N.)
Associate Professor,
Department of Radiologic Sciences,
College of Health Sciences,
Las Vegas, Nevada

CYNTHIA McCAULEY, M.Ed., R.T.(R.)
Assistant Director, Radiology,
Columbia East Houston Medical Center,
Houston, Texas

LEONARD NAEGER, Ph.D.
Professor of Pharmacology,
St. Louis College of Pharmacy,
St. Louis, Missouri

ANDREW P. WOODWARD, M.A., R.T.(R.), A.R.R.T.
Department Head,
Radiologic Technology,
WOR-WIC Community College,
Salisbury, Maryland

JAMES ZWEIG, B.S., R.T.(R.)
Director,
Radiography and Medical Imaging,
Department of Allied Health,
Clarkson College,
Omaha, Nebraska

To the two loves of my life—
Jesus Christ and **Catherine (W.W.) Jensen.**
S.J.

To the Lord, **Jesus Christ**
who bestows the tools necessary for medical miracles
to my mother, **Carol Eaton**
for all your countless hours of work and love when providing
for three children in the hardest of times

to my stepfather, **Jim Eaton**
for coming into our lives when you did

to my brother, **T.Sgt. Martin Peppers**
and sister, **Joan Denman**
for just being there in times of need

to my wife, **Kimberly**
for putting up with me

and to my twin children, **Brooke** and **Brittany**
for whom there is no greater love than
the love this father has for them!
M.P.

Preface

Our intent in writing this textbook is to help students in the medical imaging professions better understand the importance of pharmacologic principles and practices in patient care. Some technologists do not become fully aware of their role in "real" patient care until they actually begin practicing their profession.

Throughout the preparation of this book, making the content as clear and understandable as possible for today's medical imaging students and practitioners was of great importance. Each chapter opens with clearly stated objectives and a list of key terms. Within the body of each chapter you will find helpful "Did you know?" boxes. There is also an "Alert!" ⚠ that is used where appropriate to bring attention to adverse reactions and toxic effects. Each chapter ends with Learning Exercises, a workbook-style section including abbreviation identification, true-false, discussion, review, matching, and multiple-choice questions.

A pharmacology textbook is never "finished." There are always new drugs, contrast media, radionuclides, and techniques on the market and new information available about existing products. The available information seems endless, and it is a tremendous challenge to acquire enough knowledge to be a safe practitioner. We have made every effort to make the content very current by including discussions of contemporary and traditional medications and contrast media, common problems, up-to-date regulations, legal issues for technologists administering drugs, and emergency pharmacology. Particular attention has been paid to intravenous introduction of contrast media, drug nomenclature, and the physiologic processes responsible for drug actions.

The mission of *Pharmacology and Drug Administration for Imaging Technologists* is to focus on essential information that technologists need to know for safe administration of drugs; to clearly present this complex subject so readers can easily understand this material; and to provide a consistent, practical format and design with illustrations and tables that will aid readers in comprehension.

Nothing teaches the imaging technologist more about pharmacology than actually giving medications to the patient. Students should approach each encounter with a patient as an opportunity to learn. As a student or practicing technologist, you should accept it as a personal challenge to learn about each medication (contrast agent, radionuclide, etc.) ordered for a patient under your care and to understand why the medication is given in that particular situation. Because pharmacology is a rapidly changing and dynamic field, we recommend that you be exposed to supplemental drug information, such as package inserts or current drug handbooks. We encourage you to develop the habit of seeking up-to-date and timely information to supplement this book in order to provide specific details that cannot be covered in a textbook.

In working with patients, you will quickly learn that medication administration is one of the most challenging components of your role as a technologist. A technologist who develops the knowledge and skills needed to competently administer medications is highly visible and will gain the respect of both patients and colleagues in the health care system. Both the responsibilities and the personal rewards are great.

We welcome your suggestions or comments on this book so that we may continue to provide a clear and useful exposition of introductory pharmacology in future editions.

Steven C. Jensen
Michael P. Peppers

Acknowledgments

I wish to acknowledge the stimulation I have received from the many students who have asked challenging questions throughout my twenty-plus years as a teacher and the support of my professional colleagues, especially Michael Grey and Rosanne Szekely at Southern Illinois University. I am grateful for the help of the editorial, production, and design staff at Mosby and specifically thank Jeanne Rowland (project starter) and Carole Glauser (project completer) for their professionalism, attention to detail, and extreme patience. As always, I owe a special debt of gratitude to my children, Matt, Jaimie, Jordan, and Emily, for their constant love and good humor and for allowing me time away from them to complete this book. Finally, my portion of this book could not have been completed without the dedication, expertise, and abilities of my wife, Cathy. She has the knack of making the complex simple and the simple enjoyable. Her proofreading and rewriting skills are evident throughout this book.

S.J.

I wish to acknowledge all the patients I have had the honor of treating, consulting for, laughing and crying with over my ten short years of clinical practice; you have taught me things that no textbook could possibly offer! I am also grateful to David Rush, Pharm.D., and Rusty Ryan, Pharm.D., for helping me break through difficult barriers early in my educational years; you had faith in my abilities and opened doors for me that were otherwise closed. I acknowledge my emergency medicine/critical care preceptors, Joseph Barone, Pharm.D., and Wesley Byerly, E.M.T.-P., Pharm.D., for instilling in me the importance of never quitting in my quest for information and the importance of maintaining compassion and human feelings for the patient, no matter what the circumstance. I wish to thank all the nurses, doctors, and pharmacists at Mineral Area Regional Medical Center in Farmington, Missouri, for their support and trust when allowing me to become involved with their patients at the clinical level. I wish to notably thank Marie LaRose, R.N., and Perry Bramhall, D.O., for being instrumental catalysts to my clinical career in the rural environment; in many ways I wish I were still there working with you. I thank Jim Hart, Pharm.D., for the confidence displayed in my abilities and for getting me started in my pharmacy career; without your help, I could not have done it! A special acknowledgment is due for Henry Cashion, R.T.(R.), Director of Mineral Area Regional Medical Center School of Radiologic Technology. Henry has an enthusiasm and passion for making certain that his students are armed with the necessary skills to take care of patients. He is years ahead of many when it comes to practical, clinical education for the radiologic technologies. In the five years that I had the honor of teaching for his program, it became very apparent to me that Henry is an individual with high standards of ethical conduct. Henry, your students are some of the brightest that I have ever had the pleasure of teaching, and it was an honor working with you. My portion of this textbook would not have been written without your foresight.

M.P.

Contents

PHARMACOLOGY AND DRUG ADMINISTRATION

for Imaging Technologists

The Role of the Imaging Professional

OBJECTIVES

At the conclusion of this chapter you should be able to:
1. Discuss the "standards of care" in the medical imaging professions.
2. List sources of "standard of care" information.
3. Determine the legal ramifications of drug administration and venipuncture for imaging professionals in your state.
4. Locate the policies for drug administration and venipuncture at the hospital or clinic where you are most often assigned.

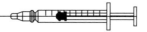

KEY TERMS

accredited program
educational standard
liability
medical malpractice
medical negligence
professional standard
scope of practice
standard of care

The physician opens the lead-lined door and steps into the brightly lit hallway. The act and its required effort were harder this time . . . it always is when one must face the family.

In the waiting room, the physician sees that the hospital chaplain has arrived and offers an all-too-familiar glance before turning to the parents. Their faces are ashen, yet it's their eyes the physician dislikes the most. For without a word being said, the dire nonverbal messages had been conveyed. "No, your daughter is not dead," the physician says. "During the examination, however, she experienced complications. She is now in a coma."

What? How? Why? These are questions that demand answers. Questions that will be answered with compassion. Both the questions and answers will never end.

"She had a seizure and went into cardiac arrest," the physician explains. "We got her back, and now hope that she'll respond further. You may see her for a few minutes. She is on a machine that assists her breathing. We're doing everything we can."

The kidney exam was necessary. Her RLQ pain and workup tests confirmed it. The IV was established. The questionnaire was completed. The patient's history of hayfever and asthma, as well as the evening hour, called for nonionic contrast. The risks were known. Radiology personnel were ready for everything . . . except for the physician's response time.

The injection went smoothly and the ER physician returned to her exceptionally busy night of accident victims and coughing infants. Following the initial film, the young female patient and the technologist were talking about the previous night's award show on television. Then the grand mal hit.

Its intensity peaked so rapidly that the RT had to grab the girl to keep her from vibrating off the table. The reaction tray was nearby, but the telephone was 10 feet away. "The emergency room is just down the hall," thought the technologist. "And the ordering ER physician knows where we are."

The patient's strength was immense. Her gurgled sounds were worse in the technologist's ears. The RT's calls for help were smothered by the enclosed room. " The "crash cart" is just outside the door," she mumbled. "So what! I wouldn't know what to give her anyway."

Then the tremors ceased as quickly as they had begun, being replaced by stillness and quiet. The RT raced to the telephone, calling the code.

INTRODUCTION

The preceding story, and far too many like it, strike fear into the hearts of many imaging professionals. In most states, medications must be prescribed by physicians or dentists. A technologist, however, may *administer* various drugs for diagnostic procedures once they are prescribed. These include medications for sedation and pain management, contrast media, and emergency drugs for reactions to contrast. Too often, the technologist (diagnostic, nuclear medicine, angiography, computed tomography, ultrasound, radiation therapy, or magnetic resonance imaging) is asked to administer these dangerous, often life-threatening drugs with little or no training in drug actions, dose calculation, methods of administration, or emergency drug therapy techniques.

HISTORICAL PERSPECTIVE

For decades, it was the responsibility of the imaging technologist to *assist* the radiologist or other physician in the administration of drug therapy. Seldom, if ever, did the technologist actually inject contrast media, sedatives, or other drugs without a physician present. The physician then remained with the patient, or within the immediate vicinity, for the duration of the examination. Times have changed. It is now common for technologists to complete examinations requiring administration of drugs to patients in settings where the physician is never present or within hailing range. As drug administration responsibilities have fallen more within the scope of practice of imaging professionals, emergency drug treatment therapies have remained only within the knowledge base of the physician.

The Joint Review Committee on Education in Radiologic Technology (JRCERT) *Standards for an Accredited Educational Program in Radiologic Sciences,* which defines radiography and radiation therapy educational practices, identifies pharmacology, patient care, and medical ethics and legal issues as required content areas for the **accredited program.** These standards do not, however, include venipuncture techniques as part of the approved curriculum. The JRCERT uses the American Society of Radiologic Technologists (ASRT) Professional Curriculum to develop and update its guidelines and standards for educational programs. In 1991, venipuncture was added to the ASRT's scope of practice description for radiographers (see box below). A logical expectation is the addition of venipuncture to the JRCERT standards for radiographers and radiation therapists.

Resolution 91-4.04. Be it resolved, that the ASRT adopt the following position statement on venipuncture: "Radiologic technologists be permitted to perform venipuncture to include the administration of contrast media, radiopharmaceuticals and/or IV medications where state statutes and/or institutional policy permits."

The Joint Review Committee on Educational Programs in Nuclear Medicine Technology identifies intravenous injections (venipuncture) as a component of the nuclear medicine technologists' scope of practice. The *Standards* of this committee specifically states: "The nuclear medicine technologist shall be able to . . . prepare and, where permitted, administer radiopharmaceuticals and other agents used in conjunction with nuclear medicine procedures to patients by intravenous, intramuscular and subcutaneous injections, aerosol and oral methods."

Additional support for the inclusion of venipuncture in the job descriptions is given by the American College of Radiology's 1987 resolution number 27. In this resolution, the ACR identifies the injection of contrast material and diagnostic levels of radiopharmaceuticals as part of the responsibilities of certified and/or licensed radiologic technologists.

ETHICAL AND LEGAL IMPLICATIONS

Review of the literature has identified conflicting information regarding which states allow technologists to perform venipuncture. A survey of officials in states requiring licensure or certification was conducted to clarify the conflicting data and to present the states' official positions relative to technologists performing venipuncture and the administration of contrast media, radiopharmaceuticals, and other drugs (see Table 1-1). *Note: At time of publication of this book, the following chart was accu-*

Table 1-1 States with Licensure or Certification Requirements

State	Nuclear Medicine	Radiography	Radiation Therapy	Is there a statement in the bill relative to technologists injecting drugs or performing venipuncture?	
				Yes	No
Arizona		X	X		X
California	X	X	X	X	
Delaware	X	X	X		X
Florida	X	X	X		X
Hawaii		X	X		X
Illinois	X	X	X	X	
Indiana		X			X
Iowa	X	X	X		X
Kentucky		X	X		X
Louisiana	X	X	X		X
Maine	X	X	X		X
Maryland	X	X	X		X
Massachusetts	X	X	X		X
Montana		X		X	
Nebraska		X			X
New Jersey	X	X	X	X	
New Mexico	X	X	X		X
New York	X	X	X	X	
Oregon		X	X		X
Tennessee		X			X
Texas	X	X	X		X
Utah	X	X	X		X
Vermont	X	X	X		X
Washington	X	X	X	X	
West Virginia		X	X		X
Wyoming	X	X	X		X

rate. *Contact your state department of health or nuclear safety for current information concerning licensure or certification.*

Only California and Georgia report that litigation has ever occurred relative to technologists injecting pharmaceuticals.

Terminology specific to venipuncture or to the intravenous administration of contrast media or other drugs for radiographers and radiation therapists (commonly defined together in state laws) was identified in six states: California, Illinois, Montana, New Jersey, New York, and Utah. All of these states, with the exception of New Jersey, provide regulations authorizing technologists to administer contrast media or other drugs, although these regulations do not necessarily authorize the technologist to perform the actual venipuncture. California and New York specifically prohibit radiographers and therapists from performing the venipuncture procedure. New Jersey prohibits these technologists from performing venipuncture and also from injecting contrast media or other drugs. Selected specific stipulations follow:

California: Radiographers and radiation therapists may ". . . assist a licensed physician or surgeon in completing an injection to administer contrast materials . . . after the performance of venipuncture or arterial puncture by a person authorized to perform those tasks. Nothing in this section shall be construed to grant technologists the authority to perform venipuncture. . . ."

Illinois: Radiographers ". . . in conjunction with radiation studies, may administer contrast agents and related drugs for diagnostic purposes."

Montana: "A radiologic technologist licensed under this chapter may inject contrast media . . . intravenously."

New Jersey: According to the Supervisor of Technologist Certification, Bureau of Radiological Health, New Jersey's Board of Medical Examiners prohibits radiographers and radiation therapists from performing venipuncture and from injecting contrast media or other drugs.

New York: "A licensed radiologic technologist may administer or inject intravascular contrast media while assisting a licensed practitioner . . . provided that . . . the licensed radiologic technologist shall not determine, directly or indirectly, the type of media to be injected or engage in the placement or insertion of the needle for intravascular media injections. . . ."

Utah: Radiologic technologists may "engage in the . . . administration of parenteral contrast media, radionuclides, and other medications incidental to radiology procedures."

All laws referring to nuclear medicine technologists include statements authorizing these technologists to apply or administer radiation, radioactive materials, radionuclides, or radiopharmaceutical agents to human beings for diagnostic or therapeutic purposes. The specific term *venipuncture,* however, is not used.

STANDARD OF CARE

In **medical negligence** (failure to do something that a reasonable person of ordinary prudence would do in a certain situation) and **medical malpractice** (breach of duty to adhere to a standard of care) cases, a **standard of care** is applied to measure the competence of the professional. The traditionally recognized standard of care required that the medical professional practice his or her profession with the average degree of skill, care, and diligence exercised by members of the same profession practicing in the same or similar locality in light of the present state of medical and surgical practice. As medicine has advanced through specialization, and as quicker and more accurate communication methods have evolved, the law has adapted and changed in most courts to disregard the previously described geographical considerations and to set the standard as that of a reasonable specialist practicing in the same field. Therefore, no matter where he or she practices, an individual practicing in the imaging sciences must maintain the same level of competence as a reasonable imaging practitioner in the same specialty.

Liability

When this principle is applied to imaging professionals, the **liability** issues increase as radiographers, nuclear medicine technologists, radiation therapists, and sonographers, depending on the limitations of state statutes and regulations, cross over specialization lines and practice in fields in which they have limited education and experience. Some states permit radiographers to perform nuclear medicine and sonographic studies as well as therapeutic procedures, nuclear medicine technologists to perform sonographic studies, and sonographers to swing back and forth across lines of specialization. Many members of these groups hold credentials in more than one field and are thereby qualified to cross lines and meet the standards of the specialties in which they practice, but a large percentage are trained on the job with limited direction and supervision.

Individuals with limited education and experience who practice as those with the appropriate education and experience will be expected to perform in the same manner as qualified personnel. A radiographer performing nuclear medicine studies will be held to the standard of a nuclear medicine technologist and not to that of a radiographer practicing nuclear medicine. Health care facilities that require employees to perform procedures beyond the employee's educational expertise will be ultimately liable for the employee, but the employee will also remain personally liable for all professional activity.

Educational Standard

The educational requirements that determine the standard of care are generally those recognized by the profession as appropriate for the field. In radiography, nuclear medicine, radiation therapy, and sonography, educational essentials have been developed that define what an accredited program must do to educate students. Curriculum guides for the imaging sciences also define specific areas of study (e.g., pharmacology and drug administration techniques) and propose appropriate content for each area. The educational essentials and the curriculum guides are periodically reviewed and revised by the JRCERT to meet the changing needs of the profession.

In cases of litigation, these educational requirements will be reviewed to determine whether a person practicing in a certain field has the requisite education. Attorneys may also review the continuing education requirements and the information available in scholarly journals and other periodicals to determine the standard of practice for a certain professional field.

The **educational standard** should be met by all personnel practicing in the field of medical imaging. Technologists and therapists should obtain and maintain certification or registration in their areas of expertise. Likewise, it is imperative that each professional understand the standard for the field in which he or she practices and maintain currency in the field by attending continuing education programs and reading pub-

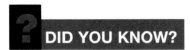

DID YOU KNOW?

Whose records are they?

Have you ever had a problem getting your medical records? Whom do they really belong to . . . the patient, the hospital, the doctor, the insurance company? They actually belong to both the patient and the clinician. The clinician (or facility) has primary custodial ownership, but the patient has proprietary rights. This means the patient has the right to reasonable access to those records, including having them transferred or seeing their contents.

lished articles and professional materials. Any professional who does not keep current and maintain continuing education places himself or herself at greater risk for both making mistakes and being liable for them.

Professional Standard

The standard established to determine the appropriate professional practice is generally that recognized by the discipline's national professional organization. The **professional standard** may be in the form of a **scope of practice,** or a series of guidelines set forth to determine what these health care specialists should and should not do under certain circumstances. Individuals practicing in these fields should be familiar with these professional requirements and should upgrade their knowledge of professional practice as the standards change and develop.

Professionals who become stagnant or refuse to change the way they practice may be personally liable if they fail to meet the recommended standards of the profession. Many believe that if they learned a procedure in school, it is the right thing to do. Reminder: just because something was learned in school does not mean it is still appropriate practice ten or twenty years later. People expect their physicians to be current in their practice, and the same is be expected of medical imaging specialists.

The imaging sciences are changing rapidly, and it is incumbent upon those who practice in these specialized fields to remain current. Inadequate time and money are generally not considered by the courts to be good reasons for being unprepared for changes in a field. Hospitals should maintain library facilities containing professional journals from many health care disciplines and offer in-service programs for employees. Public libraries carry the same or similar periodicals, and educational programs are required to maintain library resources, which are usually available to members of the profession.

The standard of care recognized by the law should be the level of care that a patient can expect and receive when entering a health care facility for professional service. When the technologist is expected to perform procedures *not* found in the professional scope of practice, it is his or her responsibility to lobby the employer for training in these procedures. The facility should then provide documentation that the employees providing these services have met minimum qualifications needed to perform them.

CONCLUSION

Although approximately one half of the states have a required certificate or licensure law, the majority of even *these* states do not specifically address venipuncture or drug administration by imaging technologists. Whether technologists in these "silent states" are protected against litigation on the basis of regional custom and tradition may be determined by the legal system. Those states with no licensure or certification laws (approximately 50%) completely expose the imaging technologist or physician and the clinical site to legal scrutiny.

Is the inclusion of a particular task in national accrediting guidelines sufficient protection against litigation, or are states responsible for this protection through specific statutory terminology? For example, is the "scope of practice" as defined by professional organizations legally protected in states where regulations conflict with national accreditation standards?

The number of technologists performing venipuncture and subsequent pharmaceutical administration is on the increase, thus also increasing the possibility of litigation against technologists. It is incumbent upon the medical imaging community to productively address these issues through increased levels of education and documented clinical competence. This book will address these issues by providing the imaging student with the background necessary to understand drug actions and classifications, administration routes and techniques, and emergency medication procedures.

Learning Exercises

Abbreviations
Spell out each of the abbreviations below.

1. JRCERT:

2. ASRT:

True-False
Circle T for true or F for false.

1. T F The American College of Radiology does not include the injection of contrast material and diagnostic levels of radiopharmaceuticals as part of the responsibilities of certified and/or licensed radiologic technologists.

2. T F It is common for technologists to administer drugs to patients without a physician present.

3. T F Scope of practice is a series of guidelines set forth to determine what health care specialists should and should not do under certain circumstances.

4. T F In a legal liability case, the courts generally recognize inadequate time and financial resources as legitimate reasons for not being familiar with changes in your specialty.

5. T F The number of technologists performing venipuncture is increasing.

6. T F A radiographer performing nuclear medicine studies will not necessarily be held to the standard of a nuclear medicine technologist rather than to that of a radiographer practicing nuclear medicine.

7. T F If a health care facility requires an employee to perform procedures beyond that employee's educational expertise, the employee is actually liable for all professional activity.

8. T F Some technologists practice across different lines of specialization, but they must hold credentials in each area of specialization.

9. **T   F**   All state laws referring to nuclear medicine technologists have statements authorizing these technologists to perform venipuncture.

10. **T   F**   The Joint Review Committee on Educational Programs in Nuclear Medicine Technology does not identify venipuncture as a component of nuclear medicine technologists' scope of practice.

Discussion Questions

1. Do you know what your state law allows medical imaging technologists to perform when administering drugs to patients?

2. What is the standard of care for your specialty?

3. In an emergency situation, what are your responsibilities? What are your limitations?

4. How would you have handled the situation described at the beginning of the chapter?

5. Where would you begin if you wanted to change your state law concerning venipuncture and drug administration?

6. What are the differences between medical negligence and medical malpractice?

7. Does your clinical facility have written guidelines concerning appropriate personnel responsible for venipuncture and drug administration?

8. Does your clinical facility assume liability for technologists who administer drugs that result in adverse reactions or death?

9. If the clinical facility does not assume the liability expressed in the previous question, do the imaging technologists continue to administer drugs?

10. How will you handle a future situation in which you are asked to administer drugs via venipuncture knowing that you are not allowed to do so under state statutes or clinical policy?

2

Principles of Pharmacology

OBJECTIVES

At the conclusion of this chapter you should be able to:
1. Define pharmacology.
2. Discuss the significance of the various names assigned to drugs.
3. Differentiate between "legend" and "over-the-counter" drugs.
4. List the seven components of a valid prescription.
5. Define controlled substance and identify the method by which controlled substances are classified.
6. Explain the significance of and methods involved in the charting of drugs and drug dosages given to patients.
7. Provide examples of questions found on patient drug histories and informed consent forms.
8. List at least five references used by health professionals to answer drug-related questions.

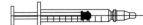

INTRODUCTION

Pharmacology is the study of drugs in living systems. It encompasses the understanding of all medication effects, whether diagnostic, therapeutic, or adverse. Drugs have led to the control or cure of many medical disorders. Yet drugs have also been responsible for many unwanted illnesses and deaths over the years. All students of pharmacology must remember that medications can be very helpful, yet can also cause serious harm to patients. No one should prescribe or administer medication without knowledge and comprehension of pharmacologic data. As a medical professional, you should learn all that you can about the potential poisons that will be placed into your patient. This book is designed to teach important principles surrounding the pharmacologic agents used frequently in the radiologic sciences.

DRUG NOMENCLATURE

A drug has many names given to it before it becomes available for use. These names include chemical name, code number, generic name, and trade or proprietary (brand) name. The generic name and the brand name are the two that most health care workers and the general public are familiar with. The other names are used primarily for research and

Chemical name — describes substance — long one (salicylic acid)
Generic Name — shortened, but still a chemical name (Asprin)

Principles of Pharmacology

manufacturing purposes. Because of the length of these other names, the **Food and Drug Administration (FDA)**—a federal government agency whose responsibility is to protect the public against fraudulent claims by manufacturers or merchants of foods or drugs—allows the name to be shortened for ease of memory. The shortened version is the generic drug name and is the official name given to the active chemical ingredient contained in a particular drug product.

Every medication has a generic name. A brand name is given to the drug by the particular manufacturer. Each manufacturer uses a different brand name for its version of the generic drug. In essence, the brand name is used as a marketing tool. The original generic drug is developed by one company. The developing company then acquires a patent for exclusive rights to manufacture and sell the generic drug as its brand drug for a specified number of years. After the patent expires, other companies may produce the same generic drug under different brand names.

For the sake of discussion, this book will refer to drugs by their generic names. In some instances, the brand name may be listed, but it will appear in parentheses after the generic name.

LEGEND DRUGS

Medications that require a prescription are called **legend drugs.** These all have a written legend (or caption) on the package stating, "CAUTION: Federal Law prohibits dispensing without a prescription." Radiopaque contrast agents and other medications administered in the radiology department fall into the category of legend drugs. The imaging technologist must therefore know what constitutes a legal prescription prior to dispensing or administering drugs or diagnostic agents ordered.

THE LEGAL PRESCRIPTION

A valid prescription or order for a drug includes at least the following seven components:
1. Patient name, room number or address, and identification numbers
2. Drug name (generic or brand)
3. Dosage (in proper units of measure for particular drug)
4. Dosage form (e.g., tablet, injection, solution)
5. Route of administration (e.g., oral, parenteral, rectal)
6. Date order is written
7. Prescriber's signature

Fig. 2-1 shows a proper hospital order sheet to be used in prescribing medication.

A prescription or order for a medication is a legal document admissible in a court of law. An important note for consideration is that a verbal order does not necessarily constitute a valid prescription. A verbal order is one that is transcribed, by a certified medical professional, to an order form or prescription form at the verbal order of the prescriber. If that prescriber does not sign that verbal order, then the prescription is

? DID YOU KNOW?

Before 1906 patent medicines and remedies were sold by medicine men in traveling wagon shows, drugstores, and mail order houses and by doctors, real or self-titled. Such products were not required to list ingredients on the label, so many contained drugs such as opium, morphine, heroin, chloral hydrate, and alcohol. Many persons (especially infants) were reportedly injured, became addicted, or died as a result of the dangerous ingredients or their quantities in these preparations.

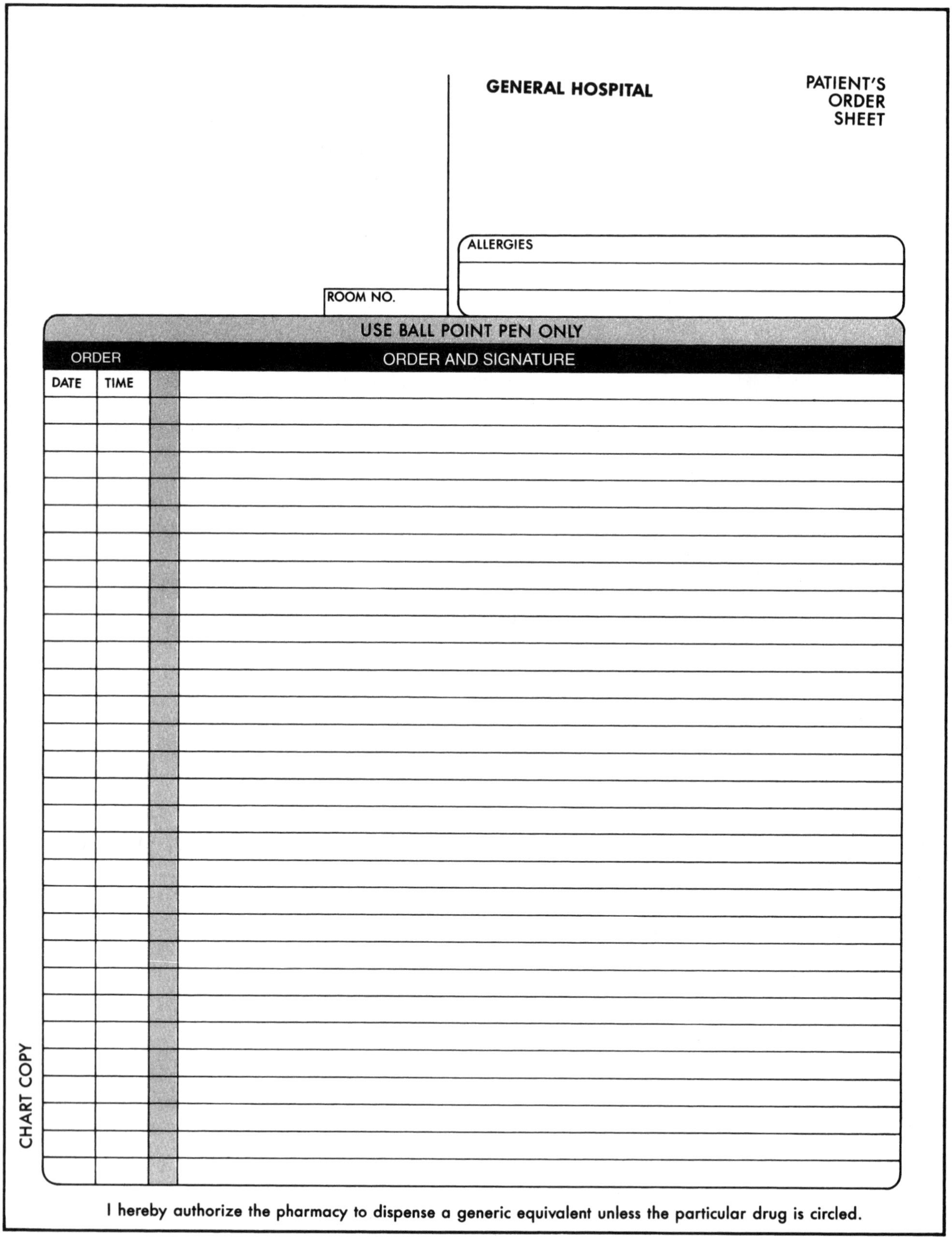

GENERAL HOSPITAL

PATIENT'S ORDER SHEET

ALLERGIES

ROOM NO.

USE BALL POINT PEN ONLY		
ORDER		**ORDER AND SIGNATURE**
DATE	TIME	

CHART COPY

I hereby authorize the pharmacy to dispense a generic equivalent unless the particular drug is circled.

Fig. 2-1 Physician's order sheet.

neither legal nor valid. It is thus in the best interests of all involved to either not take verbal orders or have in place a written protocol (to be discussed in detail in later chapters) that has been accepted as proper and standard medical care for all patients admitted to the radiology department. The protocol should be signed by all prescribers and department managers, and then placed in a safe filing system for retrieval. It should be updated on an annual basis at minimum. By preparing such a document, the imaging professional can safeguard his or her legal rights in the event of unscrupulous activity, which unfortunately can occur.

CONTROLLED SUBSTANCES

Medications that have a high potential for abuse are generally placed into one of five **controlled substance schedules.** Drugs of this nature include the **narcotic** pain relievers such as morphine, meperidine, codeine, hydromorphone, hydrocodone, pentazocine, propoxyphene, methadone, fentanyl, alfentanyl, and other opiate analogs. Also included are the sedative/hypnotic and antianxiety drugs such as chloral hydrate and benzodiazepines (diazepam, lorazepam, midazolam, temazepam, halazepam, flurazepam, triazolam, oxazepam, chlordiazepoxide, etc.). Stimulant medications such as cocaine and amphetamines are also classified as controlled substances.

Controlled substances all have a stamp placed onto the outside of the container to show which schedule they fall into. The schedules used in the United States are C-I, C-II, C-III, C-IV, and C-V. The "C" stands for controlled substance, and the Roman numeral describes the potential for abuse; the *lower* the Roman numeral, the *greater* the potential for abuse. Table 2-1 describes the potential for abuse for controlled substances as outlined using the C-I through C-V schedules.

Schedule C-I drugs are illegal for patient use in the United States. To acquire these drugs, an institution must be registered with the federal **Drug Enforcement Agency (DEA)** as either a manufacturer or a researcher of narcotic and dangerous drugs.

Schedule C-II drugs are legal for prescription use in patients and thus have the highest potential for abuse. Generally, these drugs cause marked euphoria with mind-altering effects. Potent narcotics such as morphine and strong stimulants such as amphetamine fall into this category. There are very strict regulations regarding the control and monitoring of drugs in this schedule. Each and every dosage unit must be accounted for. If counts are inaccurate by as little as one dosage unit, a report must be filed with the state agency, such as the **Bureau of Narcotics and Dangerous Drugs (BNDD),** responsible for controlling these medications. Anyone who has the responsibility to dispense or administer this schedule of medication should store the drugs under double lock and key (a locked cabinet inside a locked room) and should require two signatures for removing the medication from the supply bin. All drugs should be accounted for at the beginning and end of each employee shift. Two employees should verify the count of each and every C-II drug in the bin. The count should agree with the previous shift count minus any medica-

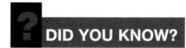
DID YOU KNOW?

The Food and Drug Act of 1906 designated *The United States Pharmacopeia* and *The National Formulary* as official standards and empowered the federal government to enforce them. Drugs were required to comply with the standards of strength and purity professed for them, and labels had to indicate the kind and amount of morphine or other narcotic ingredients present.

Table 2-1 Controlled Substance Schedules

C-I	High abuse potential. No currently accepted medical use in the United States of America. Safety for use not acceptable, even under medical supervision. Heroin, opium, lysergic acid diethylamide (LSD), marijuana ("pot"), crack cocaine, methamphetamine ("ice"), peyote buttons, mescaline, etc.
C-II	High abuse potential. Accepted medical uses under medical supervision. May lead to severe psychological and/or physical dependence. Cocaine HCl flakes, morphine, meperidine, hydromorphone, fentanyl, sufentanyl, oxymorphone, oxycodone, secobarbital, pentobarbital, etc.
C-III	High abuse potential, but less so than C-I and C-II. Accepted medical use under medical supervision. Moderate to low psychological and/or physical dependence. Acetaminophen with codeine, butalbital with caffeine and aspirin, etc.
C-IV	Abuse potential lower than C-III. Accepted medical use under medical supervision. Limited and low psychological and/or physical dependence. Diazepam, lorazepam, oxazepam, midazolam, temazepam, chloral hydrate, chlorazepate, etc.
C-V	Abuse potential lower than C-IV. Accepted medical use. Some states allow over-the-counter purchasing, provided that the pharmacist has the patient sign a register. Limited psychological and/or physical dependence. Acetaminophen with codeine cough syrup, diphenoxylate with atropine sulfate tablets, etc.

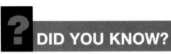
(handwritten notes: "more addicting"; "illegal for pt. use in US")

DID YOU KNOW?

International control of drugs legally began in 1912 when the first "Opium Conference" was held at The Hague. International treaties were drawn up legally obligating governments to (1) limit to medical and scientific needs the manufacturing of and trade in medicinal opium, (2) control the production and distribution of raw opium, and (3) establish a system of governmental licensing to control the manufacture of and trade in drugs covered by the convention.

tions that have been administered to patients. If the count is not correct, an investigation must take place immediately to determine why.

Schedules C-III, C-IV, and C-V drugs are also legal for prescription use. Although these medications have high potential for abuse, they are less addictive than the C-I and C-II drugs. In the health care setting, these medications should also be verified in count at the beginning and end of each shift. Storing them under double lock and key is also recommended.

CHARTING

The patient chart is a legal medical record belonging to the hospital. **Charting** should tell an accurate, chronologic history of events as they occur under the supervision of medical professionals. Members of all medical disciplines rely on the accuracy and input of others when looking through the chart. As an imaging technologist, you should respect this document and comply with the institutional procedures when entering information into the chart. This document is retained when the patient is discharged and will be used for various functions, such as patient and insurance billing, auditing, research, epidemiology, readmission information, and legal affairs. Most medical records or charts are arranged in a format to include a summary sheet, legal consents and advanced directives, a history and physical examination sheet, a problem list, physician orders, progress notes, graphic records (i.e., blood and urine results), laboratory tests, and consultations. Most hospitals use a problem-oriented medical record (POMR) format. Figs. 2-2 through 2-11 show various forms and records found in such a format.

GENERAL HOSPITAL

Patient ID Number: 437-56-5268 **Admitting date:** Sept. 16, 19••

NAME: YOUNG, Edward SEX: M MOTHER'S BIRTH NAME: Wilson

BIRTHDATE: 6-16-•• AGE: 47 TELEPHONE: 301-555-5555

ADDRESS: 1234 Flamingo Path Ellicott City, Maryland 21043

ATTENDING PHYSICIAN: J. Smarts SERVICE: Medical 4 East

ADMITTING DIAGNOSIS: Peptic ulcer

INSURANCE: Blue Cross-Blue Shield High Option

Fig. 2-2 Chart summary sheet.

GENERAL HOSPITAL

Problem Number	Date Onset	Date Recorded	Description	Status Active Inactive

Fig. 2-3 Problem list.

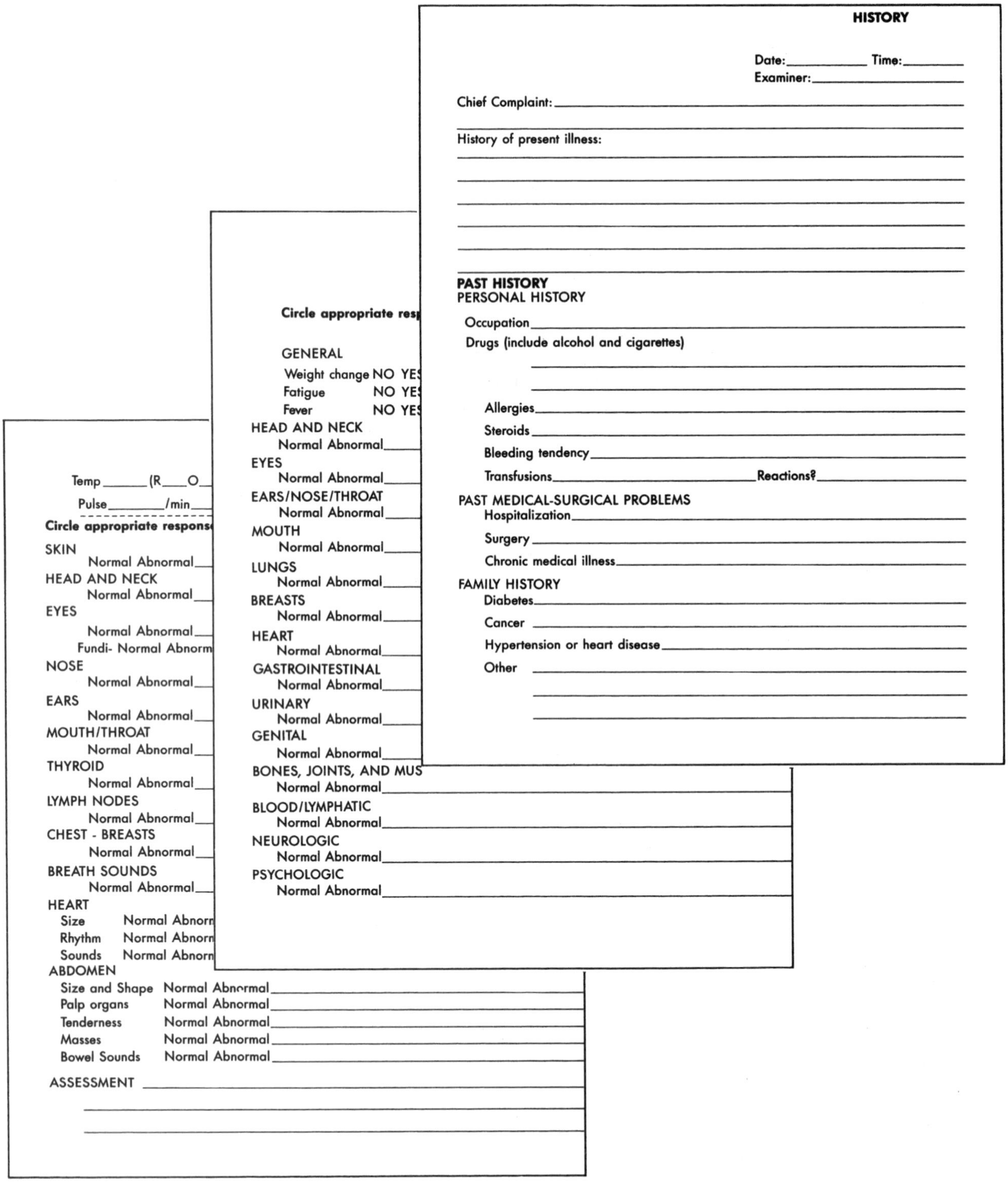

HISTORY

Date:_____ Time:_____

Examiner:_____

Chief Complaint:_____

_____

History of present illness:

_____

_____

_____

_____

_____

_____

PAST HISTORY
PERSONAL HISTORY

Occupation_____

Drugs (include alcohol and cigarettes)

_____

_____

Allergies_____

Steroids_____

Bleeding tendency_____

Transfusions_____Reactions?_____

PAST MEDICAL-SURGICAL PROBLEMS
Hospitalization_____

Surgery _____

Chronic medical illness_____

FAMILY HISTORY
Diabetes_____

Cancer _____

Hypertension or heart disease_____

Other _____

_____

_____

Circle appropriate res

GENERAL

Weight change NO YE

Fatigue   NO YE

Fever   NO YE

HEAD AND NECK

Normal Abnormal____

EYES

Normal Abnormal____

EARS/NOSE/THROAT

Normal Abnormal ____

MOUTH

Normal Abnormal____

LUNGS

Normal Abnormal____

BREASTS

Normal Abnormal____

HEART

Normal Abnormal____

GASTROINTESTINAL

Normal Abnormal____

URINARY

Normal Abnormal____

GENITAL

Normal Abnormal____

BONES, JOINTS, AND MUS

Normal Abnormal____

BLOOD/LYMPHATIC

Normal Abnormal____

NEUROLOGIC

Normal Abnormal____

PSYCHOLOGIC

Normal Abnormal____

Temp_____(R____O_

Pulse_____/min__

Circle appropriate response

SKIN

Normal Abnormal____

HEAD AND NECK

Normal Abnormal____

EYES

Normal Abnormal____

Fundi- Normal Abnorm

NOSE

Normal Abnormal____

EARS

Normal Abnormal____

MOUTH/THROAT

Normal Abnormal____

THYROID

Normal Abnormal____

LYMPH NODES

Normal Abnormal____

CHEST - BREASTS

Normal Abnormal____

BREATH SOUNDS

Normal Abnormal____

HEART

Size   Normal Abnorn

Rhythm   Normal Abnorn

Sounds   Normal Abnorn

ABDOMEN

Size and Shape Normal Abnormal____

Palp organs   Normal Abnormal____

Tenderness   Normal Abnormal____

Masses   Normal Abnormal____

Bowel Sounds   Normal Abnormal____

ASSESSMENT _____

_____

_____

Fig. 2-4   Patient history and physical examination forms.

GENERAL HOSPITAL PATIENT PROGRESS NOTES FOR NURSES AND PHYSICIANS		
Date	Time	Comments

Fig. 2-5 Patient progress notes.

GENERAL HOSPITAL CONSULTATION REPORT		
Date	Consultation record of	Service

Fig. 2-6 Consultation report.

GENERAL HOSPITAL GRAPHIC RECORD OF LABORATORY TESTS								
DATES								
WBC								
Neutrophil								
Eosinophil								
Basophil								
RBC								
HBG								
Hct								
Uric acid								
Glucose								
Sodium								
Potassium								
Chloride								
BUN								

Fig. 2-7 Laboratory test record.

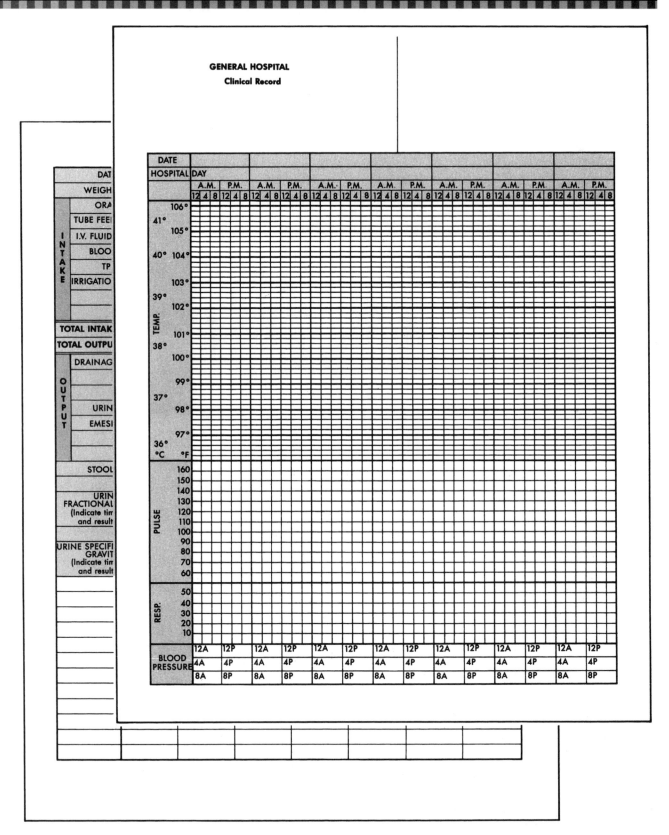

Fig. 2-8 Clinical record.

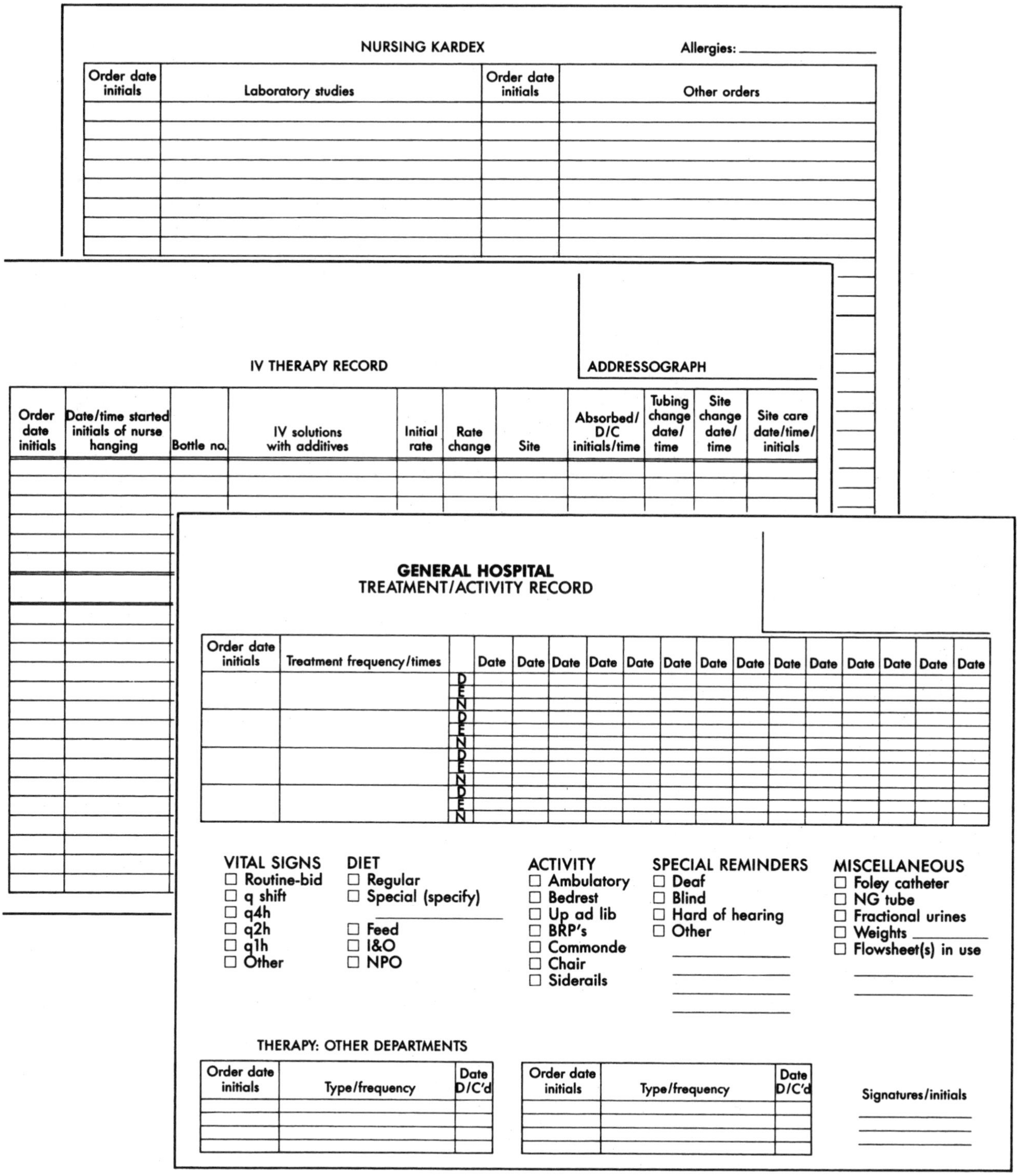

NURSING KARDEX   Allergies: _____

Order date initials	Laboratory studies	Order date initials	Other orders

IV THERAPY RECORD   ADDRESSOGRAPH

Order date initials	Date/time started initials of nurse hanging	Bottle no.	IV solutions with additives	Initial rate	Rate change	Site	Absorbed/ D/C initials/time	Tubing change date/ time	Site change date/ time	Site care date/time/ initials

GENERAL HOSPITAL
TREATMENT/ACTIVITY RECORD

Order date initials	Treatment frequency/times	D E N	Date	Date	Date	Date	Date	Date	Date	Date	Date	Date	Date	Date	Date
		D E N D E N D E N													

VITAL SIGNS
☐ Routine-bid
☐ q shift
☐ q4h
☐ q2h
☐ q1h
☐ Other

DIET
☐ Regular
☐ Special (specify) _____
☐ Feed
☐ I&O
☐ NPO

ACTIVITY
☐ Ambulatory
☐ Bedrest
☐ Up ad lib
☐ BRP's
☐ Commonde
☐ Chair
☐ Siderails

SPECIAL REMINDERS
☐ Deaf
☐ Blind
☐ Hard of hearing
☐ Other

MISCELLANEOUS
☐ Foley catheter
☐ NG tube
☐ Fractional urines
☐ Weights _____
☐ Flowsheet(s) in use

THERAPY: OTHER DEPARTMENTS

Order date initials	Type/frequency	Date D/C'd	Order date initials	Type/frequency	Date D/C'd	Signatures/initials

Fig. 2-9   Kardex treatment/activity record.

MEDICATION KARDEX

PRN MEDICATIONS

Order date initials	Expir. date	Medication dose/frequency/route		Doses given
			Date	
			Time	
			Initials	
			Date	
			Time	
			Initials	
			Date	
			Time	
			Initials	
			Date	
			Time	
			Initials	
			Date	
			Time	
			Initials	
			Date	
			Time	
			Initials	
			Date	
			Time	
			Initials	
			Date	
			Time	
			Initials	
			Date	
			Time	
			Initials	
			Date	
			Time	
			Initials	
			Date	
			Time	
			Initials	

IM Injection Site Code

1. Rt. posterior gluteal
2. Lt. posterior gluteal
3. Rt. anterior gluteal
4. Lt. anterior gluteal
5. Rt. anterolateral thigh
6. Lt. anterolateral thigh
7. Rt. deltoid
8. Lt. deltoid

Indicate the number of the site used with each IM dose given.

Record site with time.

Signatures/Initials

ALLERGIES________ DIAGNOSIS________

ROOM NO.______ NAME________ DOCTOR________ AGE______

Fig. 2-10 Medication Kardex.

GENERAL HOSPITAL

NARCOTIC INVENTORY FORM

MEDICATION: Demerol prefilled tubex Dosage: 100 mg

Number	Date	Time	Patient's name	Room	Nurse
10					
9					
8					
7					

Fig. 2-11 Narcotic inventory form.

The imaging technologist is responsible for placing various documents into the medical record. These include the specific radiologic procedure and medication orders, **informed consents** for the various procedures and medications, **patient history** regarding radiologic procedures, patient assessment during and after procedures, and any medication administration performed. (Routes and techniques of drug administration will be discussed in detail in later chapters.) Nursing and physician charting forms can be modified to fit the radiology department. The boxes on p. 24 provide examples of important documents that should be in the radiology department chart.

DRUG REFERENCES

All health care professionals should have a library of useful **drug references** to help answer any questions that may arise. For most pharmacologic questions, a combination of the following references can be used.

Physician's Desk Reference (PDR) is a general reference that is simply a compilation of various package inserts put out by pharmaceutical manufacturers. Only the FDA-approved uses and labeling are allowed to be printed. Manufacturers pay for their drugs to be listed in this reference. The *PDR* is a good reference for finding phone numbers of the major pharmaceutical companies, which are a valuable resource for information. It is important to note that the *PDR* does not necessarily contain current information on all drugs. In fact, *it does not contain all drugs.* However, it is a reference that is highly recommended because most physicians use it. The *PDR* is updated once per year.

Facts and Comparisons is available in loose-leaf and bound versions. The loose-leaf three-ring binder is recommended because the quarterly updates provided can be easily inserted into the manual. This reference is moderately extensive and concisely written, with multiple tables. The format of the text is good for quick reference, ease of use, and comprehensiveness.

American Hospital Formulary Service Drug Information is one of the most comprehensive reference books with regard to drug information. It is updated quarterly and published in full text yearly. This book, along with *Facts and Comparisons,* is considered by many pharmacists to be the reference to have for almost all questions regarding approved and nonapproved uses for drugs. The book is extensively referenced under separate cover; however, the references are available only upon request, because of the sheer volume of text required for them.

Mosby's GenRx provides comprehensive and objective prescribing information on virtually all FDA approved prescription drugs, including generic, brand, and international brand name drugs. The database of drug information is available in a variety of print and electronic formats. It also includes a full color identification section of capsules and tablets, valuable cost comparisons, unlabeled uses, cost of therapy, FDA bioequivalency ratings for generic substitution, managed care formulary coverage, and other hard-to-find drug information.

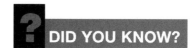

DID YOU KNOW?

The multibillion dollar pharmaceutical industry is constantly screening substances with potential marketability as new drugs. Prospective drugs may take years and huge amounts of money to progress through the FDA testing sequence listed below.

A. Animal studies, to ascertain
  1. Toxicity
    a. Acute toxicity—as determined by the **LD_{50}** (dose lethal to 50% of the animals); also known as the median lethal dose
    b. Subacute toxicity
    c. Chronic toxicity
  2. **Therapeutic index**—the ratio of the median lethal dose to the median effective dose
  3. Modes of absorption, distribution, metabolism, and excretion
B. Human studies
  1. Phase I—initial pharmacologic evaluation
  2. Phase II—limited controlled evaluation
  3. Phase III—extended clinical evaluation

EXAMPLE OF A PATIENT HISTORY PRIOR TO RADIOLOGIC EXAM

1.	Have you ever been given intravenous dye (contrast)?	YES	NO
2.	Have you ever had a bad reaction to intravenous dye (contrast)?	YES	NO
3.	Have you ever had a bad reaction to iodine?	YES	NO
4.	Do you have any allergies to medicine or vitamins?	YES	NO

4. (IF YES TO #4, PLEASE DESCRIBE_____)

5. Do you have any allergies to iodine? YES NO
   (IF YES TO #5, PLEASE DESCRIBE_____)

6. Do you have any allergies to food? YES NO
   (IF YES TO #6, PLEASE DESCRIBE_____)

7. Do you have any other allergies whatever? YES NO
   (IF YES TO #7, PLEASE DESCRIBE_____)

8. Are you pregnant or is there a possibility of pregnancy? YES NO
9. Do you suffer from sickle-cell anemia? YES NO
10. Do you feel frightened when placed in small spaces? YES NO
11. Do you have diabetes? YES NO
12. Do you have heart disease (describe_____)? YES NO
13. Do you have uncontrolled high blood pressure? YES NO
14. Do you have thyroid problems? YES NO
15. Do you have any kidney or bladder problems? YES NO
    (IF YES TO #15, PLEASE DESCRIBE_____)
16. Please list all medications you are currently taking.

_____

EXAMPLE OF A PATIENT INFORMED CONSENT PRIOR TO RADIOLOGIC EXAM WITH A RADIOPAQUE INTRAVENOUS CONTRAST AGENT

Patient Consent for Intravenous Radiopaque Contrast Enhanced CT Scan

Patient name: _____ Age: _____ Room: _____

Your physician, _____, has asked the Radiology Department to perform a test that requires the use of a radiopaque contrast agent to help in diagnosing a health problem that you may have. This test will require that the Radiology Department inject a dye (contrast media) into your vein. This dye contains iodine. If you have any known allergy to iodine or if you have ever had a reaction of any sort following a procedure requiring x-rays, CT scans, or MRI exams, then you *must* notify the technologist of this fact. If you are pregnant or could possibly be pregnant, you *must* notify the technologist.

This test and the drugs used in this test have been associated with some adverse effects, including nausea, vomiting, facial flushing, a feeling of warmth all over the body, rashes, hives, metallic taste in the mouth, allergic reactions, shock, and death. Although reactions are treatable and rare, they can occur.

I have read and understand the above information. I understand that the possible reactions that can occur include anything from nothing to death. Knowing such, I do give my consent for the Radiology Department to perform this test.

_____ /_____   _____ /_____
(signature/date)   (signature of relative/date)

Procedure explained by:

_____ /_____
(radiologist's or technologist's signature/date)

Handbook on Injectable Drugs is a comprehensive textbook that discusses physical and chemical stability of injectable drugs when combined with one another in the same intravenous tubing or syringe. It is a book that all hospital and infusion pharmacies should maintain and update for questions regarding parenteral (bypassing the gastrointestinal tract) drug products.

Drug Interaction Facts and *Hansten's Drug Interactions* are invaluable in determining whether a drug-to-drug interaction may occur when combination therapy is used.

Drugs in Pregnancy and Lactation is highly recommended in any practice that deals with pregnant patients or women who breast feed their children.

Other drug reference sources that should not be overlooked include the pharmacist, poison control centers, and computer drug information sources such as MicroMedex Drug Information, Iowa Drug Information Service, and Medline.

Learning Exercises

Abbreviations

Spell out each of the abbreviations below.

1. AHA: *American Hospital Association*

2. AHFS: *Am. Hospital Formulary Service*

3. BNDD: *Bureau of Narcotics + Dangerous Drugs*

4. DEA: *Drug Enforcement Agency*

5. FDA: *Food + Drug Administration*

6. PDR: *Physicians Desk Reference*

7. POMR: *Problem Orientated Medical Record*

True-False

Circle T for true and F for false.

1. **(T)** F   Pharmacology includes the understanding of all diagnostic, therapeutic, or adverse effects of medications in living systems.

2. T **(F)** Not all medications have a generic name.

3. T **(F)** Legend drugs do not require a prescription.

4. **(T)** F   Radiopaque drugs are considered legend drugs.

5. T **(F)** The expiration date of a drug is considered one of the seven vital components of a valid prescription or order.

6. **(T)** F   Controlled substances should be verified in count at the beginning and end of each shift.

7. T (F) Schedule C-V drugs are illegal for patient use in the United States.

8. (T) F The therapeutic index is the ratio of the median lethal dose to the median effective dose.

9. T (F) Imaging technologists are not required to place informed consent forms in the patient's chart.

10. (T) F A prescription for a medication is a legal document admissible in a court of law.

11. (T) F Manufacturers pay to have their drugs listed in the *Physician's Desk Reference (PDR)*.

Review Questions

1. Controlled substances in the United States are categorized into schedules C-I through C-V. For what does the "C" stand?

   Controlled substance

2. Does a C-I drug have a greater or lesser potential for abuse than a C-V drug?

   Greater

3. What are the two general phases of the FDA prospective drug testing sequence?

   Animal Studies + Human Studies

4. What are four useful drug references available to help with most pharmacologic questions?

   PDR, Facts + comparisons, AHFS Drug, Mosbys's Gen Rx

5. What are at least five of the documents the imaging technologist is responsible for placing into the patient's medical record (chart)?

Med Name, Date, Dose, Root, time, Tech's initials

6. What are the seven components of a valid drug prescription?

Pt.'s name, date, orders written, medication name, dosage, root, frequency of dose, prescriber's signature

Multiple-Choice Questions

Place a check before the letter of the correct answer.

1. What is the official name given to the active ingredient found in a particular drug product?
   ____ **a.** Generic name
   ____ **b.** Trade name
   ____ **c.** Code name
   ____ **d.** Chemical

2. What government agency is responsible for protecting the public against fraudulent claims by drug manufacturers?
   ____ **a.** Drug Enforcement Agency
   ____ **b.** Food and Drug Administration
   ____ **c.** Bureau of Narcotics and Dangerous Drugs
   ____ **d.** American Hospital Association

3. What is the term for medications that require a prescription?
   ____ **a.** Narcotics
   ____ **b.** Amphetamines
   ____ **c.** Nonproprietary drugs
   ____ **d.** Legend drugs

4. Which of the following controlled substance schedules contains drugs with the highest potential for abuse?
   ____ **a.** C-I
   ____ **b.** C-II
   ____ **c.** C-IV
   ____ **d.** C-V

5. Which of the following terms describes the study of drugs in living systems?
   _____ **a.** Biology
   _____ **b.** Physiology
   _____ **c.** Pharmacology
   _____ **d.** Pharmacokinetics

6. To whom does the patient chart actually belong?
   _____ **a.** Patient
   _____ **b.** Hospital
   _____ **c.** Physician
   _____ **d.** Insurance company

3

Biopharmaceutics and Pharmacokinetics

KEY TERMS

absorption
active transport
biopharmaceutics
buccal
capsule
dissolution
dosage form
emulsion
lipophilicity
parenteral
passive diffusion
pharmacokinetics
solution
sublingual
suspension
tablet
troche

OBJECTIVES

At the conclusion of this chapter you should be able to:
1. Define the key words used in describing biopharmaceutics and pharmacokinetics.
2. List the dosage forms used to deliver drug therapy.
3. Discuss the manner in which drugs are absorbed, distributed, metabolized, and eliminated in the body.

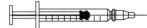

INTRODUCTION

For a drug to produce pharmacologic effects upon a body system, it must first reach the site of action. The physiochemical process a drug undertakes in reaching this site is best described via the principles of biopharmaceutics and pharmacokinetics. Think of it this way: in order to enjoy your vacation, you have to get there first. Biopharmaceutics and pharmacokinetics are analagous to what you pack, which car you take (sports car or minivan), the gas you buy on the way, and the road you take to get there. If we keep that in mind, some of the "rough spots in the road" will be easier to understand.

BIOPHARMACEUTICS

Biopharmaceutics is the area of pharmacology that focuses on the method for achieving effective drug administration. Drugs are placed into vehicles by the manufacturing process. A drug *vehicle* is a substance into which a drug is compounded for initial delivery into the body. **Dosage form**—that is, solid, liquid, gas, or any combination thereof—is the expression generally used to denote the drug and the vehicle combined. A dosage form must be capable of releasing its contents so that the drug can be delivered to the site of action. Tables 3-1 and 3-2 list various dosage forms for drug delivery.

Dosage Forms

Solid dosage forms used for oral administration include tablets, capsules, and troches. A **tablet** generally consists of an active ingredient (drug),

Table 3-1   Liquid Dosage Forms

Solution	A homogenous mixture of solid, liquid, or gas dissolved in another liquid. The solute (drug) is dispersed in the solvent (vehicle).
Emulsion	A dosage form consisting of two immiscible liquids. One liquid appears as globules uniformly dispersed throughout the other liquid. Generally, an emulsifying agent is required to maintain globule stability.
Suspension	A solid medication dispersed throughout a liquid medium. A suspending agent is generally added to help maintain uniform dispersion. Suspensions generally require agitation (shaking) prior to administration.

Table 3-2   Solid Dosage Forms

TABLETS

Compressed
Sugar coated
Film coated
Enteric coated
Multiple compressed
Controlled release
Effervescent
Buccal or sublingual

CAPSULES

Hard gelatin
Soft gelatin

TROCHES

Lozenge
Pastille

SUPPOSITORY OR INSERT

Rectal
Vaginal

various fillers and disintegrators, dyes, flavoring agents, and an outside coating; and, believe it or not, each of these things really does have a purpose. Fillers help the powdered mass to maintain form when compressed in the manufacturing process. Disintegrators aid in chemical disintegration when subjected to fluids or temperature changes. The disintegration process is required for the solid to become a solution prior to absorption across a biologic membrane. If something is not done to make it dissolve, it will come out in the same lump it went in as. Dyes and flavoring agents help make the dosage form palatable, so you can inform your kids, "It's a yummy cherry flavor." The coating may help with palatability and/or aid in the drug-releasing process.

Various types of tablets are produced to aid in the delivery of medication. *Compressed* tablets are compacted with no special coating; they are subject to chemical degradation from the environment. *Sugar-coated* tablets have a thin layer of sugar coating designed to mask bad taste and to protect the active ingredients from chemical oxidation. *Film-coated* tablets have a thin coating of material other than sugar. This type of coating serves the same function as a sugar coating, but is less expensive to manufacture. *Enteric-coated* tablets are designed to pass through the gastric area and release the active ingredients into the small intestine. This technology is used to prevent the strongly acidic contents of the stomach from chemically destroying the activity of a drug. Enteric coating is also used to prevent gastric upset by a drug known to cause significant local irritation in the stomach. *Multiple-compressed* tablets and *controlled-release* tablets are both designed to mask taste, protect contents against chemical oxidation, and allow for periodic release of contents in a controlled fashion throughout the gastrointestinal transit. Many drugs used for maintenance therapy, such as cardiovascular, pulmonary, antiepileptic, and antirheumatic medication are formulated this way to allow for once or twice daily dosing to improve patient compliance. *Effervescent* tablets contain sodium bicarbonate and an organic acid such as citrate or tartrate. These tablets liberate carbon dioxide and disintegrate into an effervescent solution in the presence of water. **Buccal** or **sublingual**

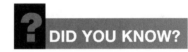

DID YOU KNOW?

Some manufacturers put surprising things in their medication that have very little to do with the primary purpose of the drug. Let's use over-the-counter analgesics such as aspirin, acetaminophin, and ibuprofen as examples. You may find one brand has two different choices, such as Supersonic Pain Killer and Supersonic Pain Killer P.M. The only difference is that the original has caffeine and the P.M. version does not. It pays to read labels.

tablets, such as nitroglycerin, are designed to disintegrate in the buccal or sublingual space and become absorbed through the buccal or sublingual vasculature.

Capsules generally consist of either a hard or a soft gelatin shell that encloses the active ingredient. A hard gelatin capsule is a two-piece shell made from calcium alginate, methylcellulose, and gelatin. A soft gelatin capsule is a one-piece shell made from similar material. Capsules are designed to mask taste, allow for ease of swallowing, and/or contribute to a controlled-release mechanism. The capsule must dissolve so that the active ingredient may be released.

Troches are generally in the form of *lozenges* or *pastilles*. These are solids that contain medicine in a hard sugar or glycerinated gelatin base designed to slowly dissolve in the mouth. Topical oral antifungals and anesthetics are most often placed in this dosage form so that continued contact will be made between the medication and the oral mucosa.

Compressed suppositories or *inserts* are solid dosage forms generally designed for vaginal or rectal delivery. Upon contact with the mucosa and in the presence of body temperature, these dosage forms melt away to release the medicinal agent.

Liquid dosage forms (Table 3-1) are used to administer medication by virtually all routes conceivable.

Parenteral dosage forms are given via injection under or through one or more layers of skin or mucous membrane. This route includes subcutaneous, intradermal, intrathecal, intracisternal, intramuscular, intravenous, and intraarterial administration. The parenteral route requires that the drug preparation be exceptionally free from all contaminants because the protective skin barrier is being bypassed. The parenteral drug vehicle is usually a solution, a suspension, or an emulsion.

Gas dosage forms are commonly used for oxygen therapy, anaesthesia, and aerosol inhalers. Oxygen is in gaseous form at room temperature and requires no dispersing agent. Most anesthetics are also gaseous at room temperature. The inhalers usually contain a liquified medication dispersed in a gas propellant such as a fluorinated hydrocarbon; upon inhaler actuation, the fluorinated hydrocarbon gas disperses the liquified medication to the bronchial system.

Disintegration and Dissolution

Medication is absorbed in either liquid or gaseous solution. Therefore, any solid or semisolid drug must first enter into one of these solution forms prior to becoming absorbed across a cellular membrane. It follows then that a medication in solid form will generally require more time to enter the body than the same medication in liquid form. Fig. 3-1 depicts the process of solid drug absorption, and the accompanying box shows the relative rapidity of absorption of various dosage forms. Disintegration and dissolution are generally considered to constitute the beginning of the pharmacokinetic process.

Absorption of Preparations

Solutions	Fastest
Suspensions	
Powders	
Capsules	
Tablets	
Coated tablets	
Enteric-coated tablets	Slowest

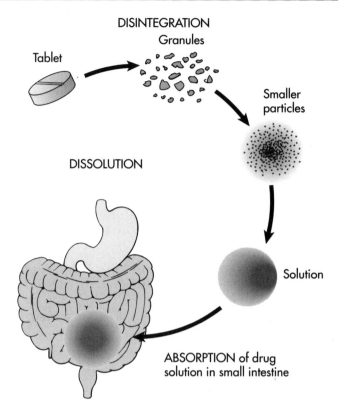

DISINTEGRATION

Granules

Tablet

Smaller particles

DISSOLUTION

Solution

ABSORPTION of drug
solution in small intestine

Fig. 3-1   Process of solid drug absorption.

PHARMACOKINETICS

Immediately upon medication administration, a drug begins to undergo the pharmacokinetic process. **Pharmacokinetics** consists of the process of how a drug is absorbed, distributed, metabolized, and eliminated throughout the body. These parameters determine the onset, duration, and extent of drug action.

Absorption

Prior to systemic action, a drug must either undergo the **absorption** process or be administered via direct intravenous injection, thus bypassing the need for absorption. Numerous anatomical sites, including gastrointestinal tract, lungs, mucous membranes, eyes, skin, muscle, and subcutaneous tissues, can be utilized for systemic drug absorption.

For absorption to occur, the physiochemical properties of the drug and the vehicle must be compatible with the site for administration. Rate and extent of drug absorption depend upon **dissolution** properties of the dosage form (previously discussed), surface area at the site, blood flow to the site, concentration of drug at the site, acid-base properties surrounding the absorbing surface, **lipophilicity** (fat-liking) of the drug, and compatibility with other chemicals or drugs.

Surface area. A large surface area allows for better absorption than does a smaller area. Pulmonary alveoli and gastrointestinal rugae give rise to some of the largest surface areas for absorption in the human body. One could compare this concept to the distance between two points. As the eagle flies, it may be five miles from point A to point B. But if you are driving in the mountains from point A to point B, you may zig-zag back and forth on a lot of hairpin curves and actually drive 25 miles. It is similar with lungs and intestines. All the "ins" and "outs" add surface area.

Blood flow. A large supply of blood frequents these sites. Blood must be flowing to the absorbing surface during the absorptive process to allow entry into the systemic circulation. Altered blood flow, as is seen in patients suffering cardiovascular shock, may change the drug absorption profile. Consequently, a patient who is in shock will generally require medication delivered via the intravenous route.

Concentration. **Passive diffusion** is the most common means by which drugs traverse cellular membranes. Drugs in solution tend to move from an area of higher concentration to an area of lower concentration. In effect, the concentration of drug at the administration site will influence both rate and extent of absorption. Fig. 3-2 depicts this process.

Exceptions to this rule include drugs that utilize an **active transport** (carrier transport) system to facilitate movement across membranes (e.g., ferrous ions). An active transport system generally contains a carrier protein to which a drug attaches. The protein complex then actively moves the drug across the membrane, then releases it on the post-absorptive side. This is like a piggyback ride with the protein doing all the work. Active transport can effectively move a drug from an area of low concentration to an area of higher concentration. Fig. 3-3 depicts this process.

Acid-base properties. Following dissolution, the *acid-base* properties of the medium in which the drug lies affect the extent of absorption across membranes. A neutrally charged, or *nonionized,* particle crosses a cell membrane better than does a charged, or *ionized,* particle. Most drugs are either weak acids or weak bases. Weak acids are nonionized in acidic mediums and ionized when in alkaline mediums. Thus, a weak acid crosses barriers best when in an acid medium.

A good example of this concept is provided by aspirin, which is a weak acid (acetylsalicylic acid). When aspirin arrives at the stomach, it enters an acidic environment where gastric juices have a pH of 1.0 to 2.0. Thus, the acidic aspirin is in an acidic environment, which makes it nonionized. This creates an easy pathway through the membrane for the drug to enter the blood. However, when a weak acid is in an alkaline environment, it becomes ionized, which hinders it from passing across cellular membranes. When the aspirin enters the blood (a slightly alkaline

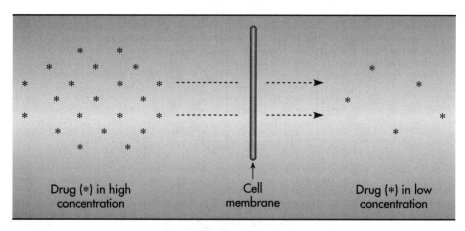

Fig. 3-2 Drug absorption via passive diffusion. The movement of drug across a cellular membrane generally occurs in the direction of highest concentration pushing toward the area in which the lowest concentration exists.

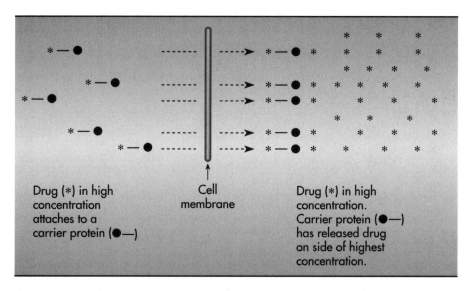

Fig. 3-3 Drug absorption via active transport. In active (carrier) transport, the movement of drug across a cellular membrane can occur in the direction of lowest concentration pushing toward the area in which the highest concentration exists.

pH of 7.4), it becomes more ionized because its pH no longer matches its environment. So, it will not cross from the blood back over into the stomach. Fig. 3-4 depicts this property of absorption.

Lipophilicity. The human cell has a double layer of lipid (fat) through which a drug must generally penetrate for absorption to occur. Drugs with good lipid solubility will cross lipid-layered membranes readily. Water-soluble drug forms will not. However, they must have some affinity for water, or they cannot dissolve and be transported by blood and other body fluids. Exceptions to this rule occur in situations

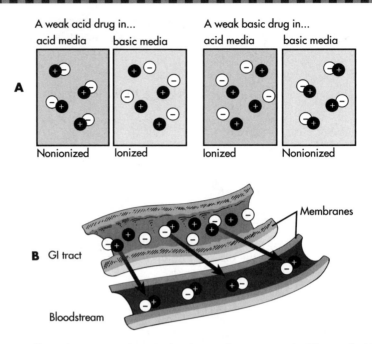

Fig. 3-4 Effect of pH upon drug ionization and transport. **A,** Effects of pH on drug molecules. **B,** Effects of pH on the transport of drug molecules through membranes.

where the human cell uses active transport, a small-pore system, or pinocytosis (the process by which extracellular fluid is taken into a cell) to allow access across the membrane.

Compatibility. Some drugs may interact with other chemicals to form insoluble precipitates. When such an interaction occurs, absorption is significantly decreased. This concept is frequently put to good use in radiologic imaging. For example, barium is extremely toxic when administered intravenously. However, barium does not cross gastrointestinal membranes well because it forms an insoluble complex (precipitate) in that medium. Thus, barium is safely used as an oral gastrointestinal radiopaque agent.

Distribution

Once a drug is absorbed into the bloodstream, it is immediately distributed throughout the body by the circulation of the blood. Distribution is defined as the transport of a drug in body fluids from the bloodstream to various tissues of the body and ultimately to its site of action. Let's use an analogy of two aspirin and trace the itinerary as we would travelers going on vacation. First, you ingest two aspirin. They begin to dissolve as soon as they contact the water and saliva in your mouth. So far, we have two travelers who leave home with their bags. The moment they get in the car, they start to get excited about their upcoming excursion. Now, they are at the airport just as the aspirin are in the stomach. The absorption that takes place in the acidic environment of the stomach is like going through the security systems at the airline gate. As soon as the aspirin hits the bloodstream, it is like stepping onto a jet going 500 mph and letting passengers parachute into all the small towns and big cities across the country. In other words, the drug goes everywhere the blood goes with two exceptions, which will be discussed later. Drug molecules are now present throughout the body just as passengers are located all over the country, but there is still one problem. The drugs must get into certain cells in order to have their desired effect. This is analogous to being forced through security systems one more time to get back into the cities. The drugs must permeate a cell membrane to get in, just as they had to permeate a cell membrane to get out (of the stomach).

Several factors affect distribution:

1. *Cardiac output:* amount of blood pumped by the heart per minute
2. *Regional blood flow:* amount of blood supplied to a specific organ or tissue
3. *Drug reservoirs:* drug accumulations that are bound to specific sites, such as plasma, fat tissue, and bone tissue

The body has two barriers to distribution made up of biologic membranes: the *blood-brain barrier* and the *placental barrier.* As one might expect, there are both advantages and disadvantages to these barriers. Given a central nervous system infection, it would be desirable to have an antibiotic that could cross the blood-brain barrier. Given an expectant mother who did not know she was pregnant, it would be undesirable for certain drugs to cross the placental barrier and affect the unborn child.

Metabolism

Drugs are taken because a certain effect is desired. However, we do not usually want that effect to last forever. Metabolism, also called *biotransformation,* chemically changes a drug into a metabolite that can be excreted from the body. The liver is primarily responsible for this task, but credit also goes to the plasma, kidneys, lungs, and intestinal mucosa.

Drugs usually undergo one or both of the following types of chemical reactions in the liver:

1. Oxidation, hydrolysis, or reduction (gaining an electron to decrease positive valence)
2. Conjugation (transforms a drug from a lipid-soluble substance that can cross biologic membranes to a water-soluble substance that can be excreted via the biliary tract)

Several factors will contribute to prolonged drug metabolism. These include liver disease, immature metabolizing enzyme systems, degenerating enzyme function, severe cardiovascular dysfunction, and renal problems.

If drug metabolism is delayed, cumulative drug effects may appear as symptoms of an overdose even though an ordinary dose was administered.

Before we leave the discussion of metabolism, one more phenomenon needs to be discussed. Drugs that are administered orally normally travel first to the liver prior to entering the general circulation. This *first-pass metabolism* may cause significant deterioration (metabolism) of the active drug, thus rendering the drug inactive. Thus, some drugs need to be administered via an alternative route to ensure the proper desired action at the intended site.

Excretion

Drug molecules, whether they are intact or metabolized, eventually must be removed from the body. This elimination is primarily accomplished by the *kidneys.* They filter the blood and remove unbound, water-soluble compounds. This is one of the reasons why drug testing is often done on urine.

The *intestines* may also eliminate drug compounds. After metabolism by the liver, a metabolite may be secreted into the bile, passed into the duodenum, and eliminated in the feces.

The third mechanism of excretion is the *respiratory system.* Gases or volatile liquids that are administered through the respiratory system usually are eliminated by the same route.

Breast milk, sweat, and saliva also contain certain drug compounds, but they are not the body's predominant mechanisms for elimination.

CONCLUSION

Drugs undergo various phases of action, which are best described using biopharmaceutical and pharmacokinetic concepts. Biopharmaceutics deals with the designing of proper vehicles and dosage forms into which a drug should be placed. The various dosage forms include solids, liquids, and gases. Drugs must first undergo dissolution prior to absorption across cellular membranes. Various physiochemical factors, including surface area of the administration site, acid-base chemistry, concentration of drug and blood flow at the absorbing surface, and the lipophilicity of the drug, may affect drug absorption. Drugs are primarily absorbed via passive diffusion, but may undergo active transport via protein carrier or utilize a pore system or undergo pinocytosis for absorption. Once absorbed, a medication is distributed to body tissues, wherein it elicits activity. Drugs are primarily metabolized by the liver and excreted by the kidneys.

Learning Exercises

Review Questions

1. Which dosage form is generally absorbed fastest, and which is absorbed slowest?

   1   Solutions

   2   Coated tablets

2. What are three factors that affect drug distribution throughout the body?

   Cardiac Output, regional blood flow, drug resevoir

3. What are three primary means of drug elimination?

   Kidneys,
   intestines, respiratory System

4. Define lipophilicity.

   - an ephinity for fat

5. What are at least four factors controlling the rate and extent of drug absorption?

   drug concentration, PH, dosage form, solubility of drug

6. What are the differences and similarities between drug absorption via passive diffusion and drug absorption via active transport?

   MAJORITY
   ↳ Movement from high concentration → L.C. to = out
   active - carriers transport drugs across membrane
   ↳ more rapid

Fill-in-the-Blank Questions

1. The _____*blood-brain barrier*_____ and the _____*placental barrier*_____ are two drug distribution barriers the body has that are made of biologic membranes.

2. _____*biotransformation*_____ is another name for metabolism.

3. _____*biopharmaceutics*_____ is the area of pharmacology that focuses on the method for achieving effective drug administration.

4. _____*pharmocokinetics*_____ includes the processes of how a drug is absorbed, distributed, metabolized, and eliminated throughout the body.

5. The most common way drugs traverse cellular membranes is _____*Passive diffusion*_____.

6. _____*active Transport*_____ can move a drug from an area of low concentration to an area of higher concentration.

7. Medications must go through disintegration and _____*dissolution*_____ in order to be absorbed across a cell membrane.

Matching

Match the following terms with the appropriate descriptive phrases.
a. Compressed tablets
b. Sugar-coated tablets
c. Film-coated tablets
d. Enteric-coated tablets
e. Capsules
f. Troches
g. Compressed suppositories
h. Parenteral dosage forms

_F_ 1. Lozenges or pastilles; topical oral antifungals
_C_ 2. Less expensive to manufacture than sugar coating
_A_ 3. Subject to chemical degradation from the environment
_E_ 4. Hard or soft gelatin encloses the active ingredient
_B_ 5. Mask taste and protect active ingredients from chemical oxidation
_D_ 6. Release medicinal agent upon contact with mucosa and melting
_G_ 7. Release active ingredients into the small intestine
_H_ 8. Injection under or through one or more layers of skin or mucous membrane

Multiple-Choice Questions

Place a check before the letter of the correct answer.
1. What is the term for the substance into which a drug is compounded for initial delivery into the body?
   _____ a. Drug dose
   _____ b. Drug vehicle
   _____ c. Drug suspension
   _____ d. Drug filler

2. How are drugs eliminated from the body?

_____ **a.** Metabolism

_____ **b.** Ionization

_____ **c.** Excretion

_____ **d.** Both a and c

3. What is the term for the most common means by which drugs traverse cell membranes?

_____ **a.** Active transport

_____ **b.** Passive diffusion

_____ **c.** Lipophilicity

_____ **d.** Cellular absorption

4. What is the general term for lozenges or pastilles?

_____ **a.** Capsules

_____ **b.** Tablets

_____ **c.** Troches

_____ **d.** Inserts

5. What is the term for the process of how a drug is absorbed, distributed, metabolized, and eliminated in the body?

_____ **a.** Pharmacodynamics

_____ **b.** Biopharmaceutics

_____ **c.** Pharmacokinetics

_____ **d.** Cellular diffusion

6. Which of the following dosage forms is designed to mask taste, allow for easy swallowing, and contribute to controlled release of the drug?

_____ **a.** Troches

_____ **b.** Tablets

_____ **c.** Pastilles

_____ **d.** Capsules

7. Which of the following drug dosage forms consists of two immiscible liquids?

_____ **a.** Solution

_____ **b.** Emulsion

_____ **c.** Suspension

_____ **d.** Parenteral

8. Which of the following drug dosage forms is a mixture of solid, liquid, or gas dissolved in another liquid?

_____ **a.** Solution

_____ **b.** Emulsion

_____ **c.** Suspension

_____ **d.** Parenteral

4 Pharmacodynamics

OBJECTIVES

At the conclusion of this chapter you should be able to:
1. List and describe the three mechanisms of drug action.
2. Explain the differences between agonistic and antagonistic drug responses.
3. Recognize and interpret a serum concentration-time profile.
4. Discuss the significance of a drug's half-life of elimination.
5. Cite and define terms associated with negative responses to drug action.

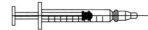

INTRODUCTION

After absorption and distribution, a drug reaches its site of action to produce an effect. *Pharmaco* refers to drugs and *dynamics* refers to what happens when two things meet and interact—that is, the drugs and your body. In essence, **pharmacodynamics** is the study of how the effects of a drug are manifested. Various terms are used in pharmacodynamics, including mechanism of action, onset of action, therapeutic effect, adverse effect, toxicity, termination of action, side effect, and allergic reaction.

MECHANISM OF ACTION

The method by which a drug elicits effects is known as the **mechanism of action.** Drugs produce effects via drug-receptor stimulation or blockade, drug-enzyme interactions, or nonspecific drug interactions.

Drug-Receptor Interactions

Receptors are specific biologic sites located on a cell surface or within a cell (Fig. 4-1). Receptors can be thought of as keyholes into which specific keys (drugs) may fit. Drugs have specific **affinity** (attraction) for their specific receptors. Strong affinity for a receptor will allow a drug to elicit an **agonist, antagonist,** or *mixed agonist/antagonist* interaction. The organ on or in which the desired effect occurs is generally called the **target organ.** The target organ can represent any organ or system in the body.

An agonist is a drug or natural substance with an affinity for specific receptor sites that produces a physiologic response, usually predictable. A

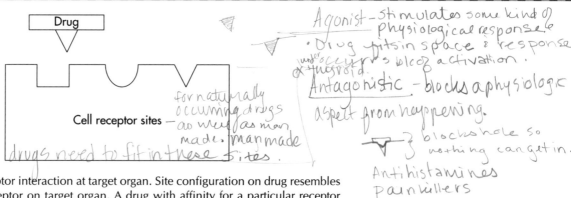

Fig. 4-1 Drug receptor interaction at target organ. Site configuration on drug resembles configuration of receptor on target organ. A drug with affinity for a particular receptor will attach to the receptor and produce an agonistic, antagonistic, or mixed agonistic/antagonistic response.

drug agonist simply stimulates or enhances the body's natural response to stimulation. An example of such activity is seen with the use of epinephrine in a patient suffering acute bronchospasm secondary to anaphylaxis. Epinephrine will stimulate a beta$_2$ receptor in the lungs to cause bronchodilation. The beta$_2$ receptor is normally stimulated by endogenous epinephrine, known as adrenaline, but the patient may not have enough of his or her own epinephrine to prevent severe respiratory distress when suffering acute anaphylaxis. By administration of epinephrine, a beta$_2$ receptor agonist, the normal physiologic function of the beta$_2$ receptor can be enhanced to stimulate bronchodilation. No new function was developed. A normal physiologic/biologic function was simply enhanced.

Think about the lock and key analogy. The endogenous epinephrine key plugs into the receptor site lock to open the door for bronchodilation to occur. The problem in acute anaphalaxis is that not enough keys are available to unlock enough doors to allow bronchodilation to stop the crisis. The epinephrine given to the patient is like pouring a lot of new keys into the bloodstream to unlock a lot more doors. Drugs with antagonist activity will block receptors for which they have affinity. The normal physiologic/biologic function carried out by the receptor cannot ensue; the door cannot be opened because the keyhole is blocked. In the example given above, a patient suffering severe anaphylaxis may have worsening respiratory distress if given the drug propranolol, a beta$_2$ receptor blocker. Propranolol acts as an antagonist to the normal function of the beta$_2$ receptor in the lungs.

Breaking the words agonist and antagonist into their parts will help to keep the two from being confused. The agonist enhances a response. The word antagonist is agonist with the prefix "ant" added, which means against. So antagonists diminish the response either of endogenous agonists or other drugs. A more complete list of definitions is given in the box on p. 44.

Drug-Enzyme Interactions

Enzymes occur throughout body systems and are generally considered catalysts responsible for bringing forth biochemical reactions. Many en-

DRUG-RECEPTOR INTERACTION TERMS

affinity the propensity of a drug to bind or attach itself to a given receptor site.

efficacy (intrinsic activity) the drug's ability to initiate biologic activity as a result of such binding.

agonist a drug that combines with receptors and initiates a sequence of biochemical and physiologic changes; possesses both affinity and efficacy.

antagonist an agent designed to inhibit or counteract effects produced by other drugs or undesired effects caused by cellular components during illness.

competitive antagonist an agent with an affinity for the same receptor site as an agonist; the competition with the agonist for the site inhibits the action of the agonist; increasing the concentration of the agonist tends to overcome the inhibition. Competitive inhibition responses are usually reversible.

noncompetitive antagonist an agent that combines with different parts of the receptor mechanism and inactivates the receptor so that the agonist cannot be effective regardless of its concentration. Noncompetitive antagonist effects are considered to be irreversible or nearly so.

partial agonist an agent that has affinity and some efficacy but that may antagonize the action of other drugs that have greater efficacy. Not infrequently, antagonists share some structural similarities with their agonists.

zymes begin working after becoming attached to a particular substrate; this is analogous to a drug attaching to a receptor. A drug-enzyme interaction occurs when a drug resembles the substrate that an enzyme usually attaches to. Stimulation or blockade of the enzyme will then occur as a result of the drug, thus producing a pharmacodynamic reaction. One example of this type of pharmacodynamic reaction is found in chemical warfare when nerve gas is used. Some nerve gases act to tie up (or block) acetylcholinesterase enzyme. Acetylcholin-esterase enzyme metabolizes acetylcholine, a neurotransmitter responsible for nerve stimulation. Inhibition of acetylcholinesterase enzyme will allow acetylcholine to accumulate, reaching toxic levels in the nervous system. After reaching toxic levels, acetylcholine will produce marked nausea and vomiting, massive diarrhea, profuse sweating, pulmonary edema, and seizures. This will progress until the drug effects on acetylcholinesterase are stopped. Another example, seen more frequently in medicine, is the cytochrome P_{450} enzyme interactions with various medications. Cytochrome P_{450} enzyme is responsible for metabolism of many medications. Any interference with this enzyme can lead to decreased metabolism with concomitant drug accumulation. Cimetidine (an antiulcer medication) is one drug that antagonizes cytochrome P_{450} very strongly. Theophylline (an antiasthmatic) is one drug that requires the enzyme for metabolism. Combining cimetidine plus theophylline can and does lead to theophylline poisoning, if not closely monitored. Since theophylline poisoning can become rapidly fatal, it should become quite apparent why it is important to understand drug-enzyme interactions.

Nonspecific Drug Interactions

Finally, some drugs may elicit pharmacologic effects via nonspecific pharmacodynamics. For example, ointments and emollients may physically block underlying tissues from the outside environment. The radiopaque contrast media, discussed in later chapters, elicit their desired effects via the radiopaque iodine contained within their structure. Some drugs penetrate cell membranes or accumulate within a cell or cavity so that interference with normal cell biochemical function occurs.

DRUG-RESPONSE RELATIONSHIPS

Two other terms need to be introduced at this point: *efficacy* and *potency.* Efficacy is the degree to which a drug is able to produce the desired effect (how great the effect will be). Potency is the relative concentration required to produce that effect (how much drug is needed). For example, if drug A produces a reduction in pain from severe to mild and drug B reduces pain from severe to none at all, drug B is more efficacious. If drug C and drug D both provide total pain relief, but you must take 5000 mg of drug C and only 200 mg of drug D, then drug D is more potent. The dynamics of these two phenomena are related to receptor-drug interaction.

SERUM CONCENTRATION-TIME PROFILE TERMS

onset of action or latent period interval between the time a drug is administered and the first sign of its effect

termination of action point at which a drug effect is no longer seen

duration of action period from onset of drug action to the time when response is no longer perceptible

minimum effective concentration lowest plasma concentration that produces the desired drug effect

peak serum concentration highest plasma concentration attained from a dose

toxic level plasma concentration at which a drug produces toxic effects

therapeutic range range of plasma concentrations that produce the desired drug effect without toxicity (the range between minimal effective concentration and toxic level)

After drug administration, the amount that reaches and remains in the systemic circulation depends upon the rates and extent of absorption, distribution, metabolism, and elimination. Fig. 4-2 is a graphic representation of response once drugs are administered. It simply shows what happens over time as indicated by the serum concentrations of a drug: the **serum concentration-time profile.**

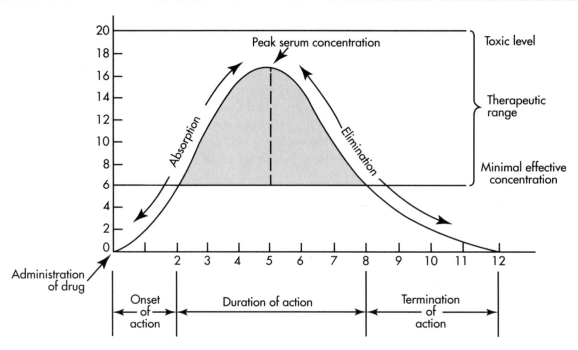

Fig. 4-2 Drug serum concentration-time profile.

HALF-LIFE

The time required for the current serum drug concentration to decline by 50% is termed the biological half-life or **half-life of elimination.** The half-life of elimination generally remains stable for each particular drug, unless metabolism and/or excretion are altered (as in septic shock). The drug dosage does not generally alter the half-life of elimination. However, there are a few drugs, such as phenytoin, aspirin, and alcohol, that may have alterations in their respective half-lives of elimination when dosages overwhelm the biologic capacity for metabolism. Fig. 4-3 uses theophylline, an antiasthma drug, to illustrate the concept of half-life of elimination.

THERAPEUTIC INDEX

The *therapeutic index* is a measure of the relative safety of a drug. It is a ratio between two mathematical factors:
1. Lethal dose (LD_{50}): the dose at which a drug is lethal to 50% of the population
2. Effective dose (ED_{50}): the dose required to produce a therapeutic effect in 50% of the population

The therapeutic index is calculated with the following formula:

$$TI = \frac{LD_{50}}{ED_{50}}$$

The closer the calculation is to 1, the more dangerous the drug is. If it takes a lethal dose to get a therapeutic effect, you may kill your patient at the same time you are trying to cure him.

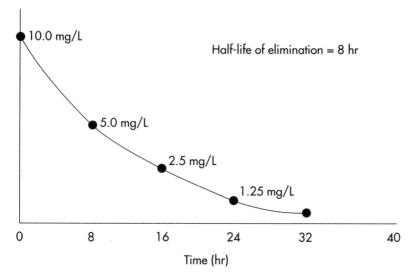

Fig. 4-3 Half-life of elimination of theophylline. Theophylline is an antiasthma drug that exhibits a half-life of elimination approximately equal to 8 hours in most individuals. Therefore, it will take 8 hours for a serum theophylline concentration of 10 mg/L to decline to 5 mg/L, provided no more theophylline enters the body. It will then take another 8 hours to decline to 2.5 mg/L, another 8 hours to decline to 1.25 mg/L, and so on. A drug requires approximately four to five half-lives of elimination to be completely cleared from the body.

ADVERSE EFFECTS

A **side effect** is generally considered a predictable pharmacologic action on body systems other than the action intended. Side effects can be either good or bad, depending on the situation. Any unwanted effect is an **adverse effect.** For example, hydroxyzine is a strong antihistamine medication that can be used to prevent itching. Two side effects of this drug are antiemetic activity and anxiety relief, both of which may be considered good but not the primary drug function. Meperidine (Demerol) causes frequent nausea and vomiting, which are adverse effects. The good side effects of hydroxyzine will lessen the adverse effects of meperidine while simultaneously relieving anxiety often associated with pain. However, another side effect of hydroxyzine is constipation, which could lead to impaction and a severely adverse outcome. Thus, all adverse effects need to be considered, and an acceptable ratio between the good and bad should be sought for all drug therapy.

Toxicity is also an extension of pharmacologic action, and is directly related to dose. The higher the dose, the greater the toxic effects. This is an area of concern for medical imaging technologists as well as you as a consumer. One must remember that a normal dose may become toxic if metabolism or elimination is impaired.

An **allergic reaction** results from an immune-mediated response by the body against the drug and is not necessarily related to dose. Both toxic and allergic effects are adverse.

Absolutely no drugs are completely safe. All have potential to cause side, adverse, toxic, and/or allergic effects in the human body. In some cases, the effects are immediately noticed; other cases require weeks to manifest the effects. Patients should never be given a medication without proper, systematic, and critical thought. Even water has killed those who have overdosed on it!

DRUG-DRUG INTERACTIONS

A **drug-drug interaction** occurs when two or more drugs act in unison to produce additive agonist, synergistic, or antagonist responses. Many drugs will alter the metabolism of other drugs, thus leading to accumulation and possible toxicity. Some drugs, such as the sedative-hypnotics, will synergize with others in their class. Synergism simply means that two drugs act together to give a pharmacologic response that is greater than the additive response expected. Alcohol plus diazepam (Valium) is a good example of a synergistic combination. The sedative properties of either drug alone may not make a person comatose at small doses. However, when alcohol is taken with diazepam, the patient may suffer severe central nervous system depression with a comatose state.

Another type of drug-drug interaction is chemical incompatibility. When two drugs of different chemical natures are placed together, they may precipitate to an insoluble complex or just chemically destroy their activity.

CONCLUSION

Pharmacodynamics is the study of the way drugs act upon the body. Drugs produce effects via drug-receptor stimulation or blockade, drug-enzyme interactions, or nonspecific drug interactions. Drugs do not confer any new biologic functions; they simply enhance or block existing functions. The serum concentration-time profile helps to illustrate onset of action, minimum effective and toxic concentrations, peak serum concentration, half-life of elimination, and duration of action. No drug is considered absolutely safe; all can exhibit adverse and potentially toxic effects. Likewise, all drugs have the potential to interact with other drugs to cause either beneficial or adverse outcomes.

DID YOU KNOW?

Concerned parents often give their children doses of drugs for a variety of reasons: cold medicines, antibiotics, etc. One of the factors that physicians, pharmacists, and pharmaceutical companies are concerned with is the therapeutic index for pediatric patients. Some drugs require an adult dose to achieve the therapeutic effect. However, children's kidneys and livers are not fully mature and able to handle the adult dose. Any medication given to a child should be responsibly and carefully considered.

Learning Exercises

True-False

Circle T for true and F for false.

1. T **F** The plasma concentration at which a drug no longer produces serious adverse effects is known as the toxic level.

2. T **F** The therapeutic index is a measure of the relative effectiveness of a drug.

3. **T** F Drugs have a specific affinity for their specific receptors on a cell surface or within a cell.

4. T **F** Half-life is the time required for the current serum concentration to double.

5. **T** F The half-life of elimination generally remains stable for most drugs.

6. T **F** Some drugs are completely safe.

7. **T** F Efficacy is the degree to which a drug is able to produce the desired effect.

8. T **F** The latent period is the point at which a drug effect is no longer seen.

9. T **F** Side, adverse, and toxic effects of drugs always are manifested immediately.

10. **T** F Radiopaque contrast media elicit their desired effects via the radiopaque iodine contained in their structure.

Fill-in-the-Blank Questions

1. Generally thought to be catalysts responsible for changes in biochemical reactions, _enzymes_ occur throughout the body systems.

2. A _side effect_ is a predictable pharmacologic action on body systems other than the action intended.

3. When two drugs are combined and cause a pharmacologic response that is greater than it would have been if the drugs had been given individually, this is known as _synergism_.

4. The method by which a drug elicits effects is known as the _mechanism of action_.

5. The organ in which the _desired effect_ occurs is generally called the target organ.

6. A _drug-enzyme interaction_ occurs when a drug resembles the substrate to which an enzyme usually attaches.

7. After drug administration the amount that reaches and remains in the systemic circulation depends on _rate + extend of absorption_, _distribution_, _metabolism_, and _elimination_.

8. Any unwanted effect from a drug is termed _adverse_.

9. Both toxic and allergic effects are known as _adverse_.

10. A _drug/drug interaction_ occurs when two or more drugs act in unison to produce additive agonist, synergistic, or antagonist responses to each other.

Multiple-Choice Questions

Place a check before the letter of the correct answer.

1. What term is defined as the study of the manner in which drug effects are manifested?
   ____ **a.** Pharmacokinetics
   ____ **b.** Pharmacodynamics
   ____ **c.** Affinity
   ____ **d.** Toxicity

2. Drugs produce effects via mechanisms of action termed drug-receptor stimulation or blockade, nonspecific drug interactions, or which of the following?
   ____ **a.** Drug-drug interactions
   ____ **b.** Physiologic/biologic processes
   ____ **c.** Drug-enzyme interactions
   ____ **d.** Pharmacologic effect

3. What is the term for specific biologic sites located on a cell surface or within a cell that attract certain drugs?
   _____ a. Target organs
   _____ b. Organelles
   _____ c. Receptors
   _____ d. Keys

4. Which of the following is true of drugs with antagonistic activity?
   _____ a. They stimulate receptors for which they have affinity.
   _____ b. They block receptors for which they have affinity.
   _____ c. They destroy receptors for which they have affinity.
   _____ d. They have no effect on receptors for which they have affinity.

5. What is the term for the catalysts responsible for bringing forth changes in biochemical reactions?
   _____ a. Proteins
   _____ b. Agonistic drugs
   _____ c. Substrates
   _____ d. Enzymes

6. What is the mechanism by which radiopaque contrast media elicit their desired effects via the radiopaque iodine contained within their structure?
   _____ a. Drug-enzyme interaction
   _____ b. Drug-drug interaction
   _____ c. Nonspecific drug interaction
   _____ d. Serum-drug interaction

7. What is the term for a predictable extension of pharmacologic action into body systems other than those intended?
   _____ a. Toxic effect
   _____ b. Side effect
   _____ c. Adverse effect
   _____ d. Allergic effect

8. Which of the following are depicted on the plasma concentration graph?
   _____ a. Onset of action
   _____ b. Toxic concentrations
   _____ c. Half-life of elimination
   _____ d. All of the above

Review Questions

1. Using the serum concentration-time profile, what is the significance of toxic serum concentration?

Dosage was higher than the required peak drug performance.

2. What are the three mechanisms of drug action?

Drug - receptor interactions

Drug - enzyme interactions

Non-specific drug interactions

3. When does a drug-drug interaction occur, and what does it produce?

When 2 or more drugs act together, that causes an antagonistic reaction or response

4. What is the relationship between dose and toxic effect?

↑ dose ↑ toxic effect also the dose may become toxic if metabolism or elimination is impared.

Classification, Chemistry, ? Pharmacology of Contras

OBJECTIVES

At the conclusion of this chapter you should be able to

1. Define radiopaque contrast media (ROCM).
2. Discuss the importance of iodine in ROCM.
3. Differentiate between osmolarity, osmolality, and osmotic activity.
4. Identify and discuss the three categories of intravascular radiopaque contrast media.
5. Cite the advantages and disadvantages of the three forms of enteral radiopaque contrast media.

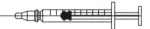

RADIOPAQUE CONTRAST MEDIA

Radiopaque contrast media (ROCM) are high-density pharmacologic agents used to visualize low-contrast tissues in the body such as the vasculature, kidneys, gastrointestinal (GI) tract, and biliary tree.

The most commonly prescribed ROCM are iodine and barium. The atomic number of iodine is 53 and the atomic number of barium is 56. Each has a much higher atomic number and mass density than the low-contrast tissues listed above. When an iodinated compound fills a blood vessel or when barium fills a portion of the gastrointestinal tract, these internal organs become visible on a radiograph. Low-kilovoltage techniques (below 80 kVp) are usually selected in order to produce high-contrast radiographs of the blood vessels or genitourinary tract. Higher-kilovoltage operation (above 90 kVp) is used in GI examinations, not only to reveal the presence of the organ but also to penetrate the contrast media to see the walls and inner structures.

PHARMACOLOGY OF IODINATED ROCM

Radiopaque contrast media are available in **parenteral** and **enteral, ionic** and **nonionic,** high-osmolality and low-osmolality forms. With the exception of barium, ROCM used for roentgenography are derivatives of **triiodinated benzoic acid** (Fig. 5-1).

Iodine molecules contained within ROCM are effective photon absorbers in the human body. The iodine molecules essentially do not allow as many photons to pass through for projection onto the radio-

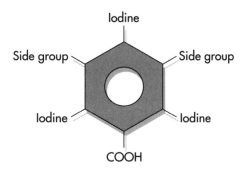

Fig. 5-1 Triiodinated benzoic acid.

graphic film. Thus, iodine molecules are responsible for the silhouette images projected. Radiopacity elicited by ROCM is a direct function of the percentage of iodine (except in the case of barium sulfate) in the molecule and the concentration of media present. In the case of barium sulfate, barium acts as iodine.

OSMOLALITY, OSMOLARITY, OSMOTIC ACTIVITY

Before discussing the intravascular ROCM, we must first understand the concepts of **osmolality, osmolarity,** and **osmotic activity.** Osmosis is the movement of water across a semipermeable membrane. The membrane must be more permeable to water than to the solute, and there must be a greater concentration of solute on one side so that water is drawn across the membrane to the side of higher solute concentration in order to equilibrate the solute concentrations.

Osmolality controls the distribution and movement of water between body compartments. The terms osmolality and osmolarity are often used interchangeably in reference to osmotic activity, but because one measures in weight and the other measures in volume, they define different measurements. Osmolality is the number of milliosmoles per kilogram of water, or the concentration of molecules per weight of water. Osmolarity is the number of milliosmoles per liter of solution, or the concentration of molecules per volume of solution. Sometimes the difference between the two measurements is insignificant. In the case of plasma, there are a number of solutes (proteins, glucose, lipids, etc.), so the difference between osmolality and osmolarity becomes more significant.

Simply stated, a highly osmotic agent will attract water so that a dilutional effect can occur to equilibrate pressures between two permeable or semipermeable membranes. Fig. 5-2 illustrates the effects of osmotically active particles in solution. Highly osmotic substances, such as ROCM, placed into the bloodstream will cause fluid from outside the bloodstream (extravascular space) to be drawn into the bloodstream (intravascular space). This effectively dilutes osmotic particles until osmotic pressures equilibrate between the intravascular and extravascular spaces. Ultimately this results in both a dilution of normal intravascular constituents (e.g., albumin, electrolytes, sugar) and an increase in in-

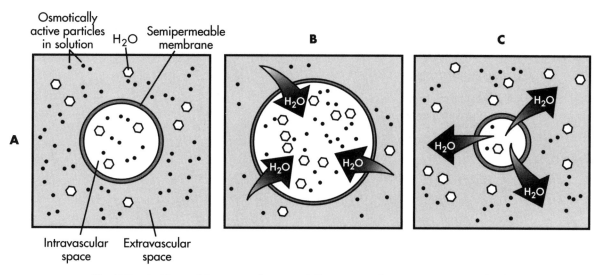

Fig. 5-2 A, Normal intravascular osmolality or osmolarity. **B,** Intravascular hyper-osmolality or hyper-osmolarity. **C,** Intravascular hypoosmolality or hypoosmolarity.

travascular hydrostatic (fluid) pressures. These osmotic influences contribute to adverse cardiac and renal effects experienced with ROCM.

INTRAVASCULAR RADIOPAQUE CONTRAST MEDIA

Intravascular (i.e., intravenous and/or intraarterial) ROCM are used to add density to vascular structures. Increased density of the media alters the attenuation of x-rays passing through the area, thus enhancing the anatomic image on the radiographic film.

Categories

Three broad categories of intravascular ROCM exist: *high-osmolality ionic ROCM, low-osmolality nonionic ROCM,* and *low-osmolality ionic ROCM.* Generally, ionic ROCM exist in salt forms consisting of sodium and/or meglumine (Tables 5-1 and 5-3), while nonionic ROCM are supplied as nonsalt forms (Table 5-2). High-osmolality ionic ROCM, such as those listed in Table 5-1, contain three iodine atoms per molecule and dissociate into two osmotically active particles when injected into the bloodstream. These particles consist of one radiopaque **anion** (negatively charged particle) and one **cation** (positively charged particle) for every three iodine atoms in solution (Fig. 5-3). These ionic ROCM are referred to as **ratio-1.5 media** because the ratio of iodine atoms to osmotically active particles is 3:2. The newer low-osmolality nonionic ROCM, such as in those listed in Table 5-2, contain three iodine atoms per molecule and do not dissociate in solution. These exist as one osmotically active particle for every three iodine atoms (Fig. 5-4) and are thus referred to as **ratio-3.0 media** (the ratio of iodine to osmotically active particles is 3:1). Finally, the newer low-osmolality ionic ROCM, such as those listed in Table 5-3, consist of six iodine atoms per molecule and dissociate into two osmotically active particles (Fig. 5-5).

Table 5-1 High-Osmolality Ionic Intravascular Radiopaque Contrast Media

	Percentage of iodine
MEGLUMINE SALTS	
Diatrizoate meglumine 30% (Hypaque Meglumine 30%) (Reno-M-Dip) (Urovist Meglumine DIU/CT)	14.1
Diatrizoate meglumine 60% (Angiovist 282) (Hypaque Meglumine 60%) (Reno-M-60)	28.0
Diatrizoate meglumine 76% (Diatrizoate Meglumine 76%)	35.8
Iodamide meglumine 24% (Renovue-Dip)	11.1
Iodamide meglumine 65% (Renovue-65)	30.0
Iodipamide meglumine 10.3% (Chlorografin Meglumine)	5.1
Iodipamide meglumine 52% (Chlorografin Meglumine)	25.7
Iothalamate meglumine 30% (Conray 30)	14.1
Iothalamate meglumine 43% (Conray 43)	20.2
Iothalamate meglumine 60% (Conray)	28.2
SODIUM SALTS	
Diatrizoate sodium 25% (Hypaque Sodium 25%)	15.0
Diatrizoate sodium 50% (Hypaque Sodium 50%) (Urovist Sodium 300)	30.0

Table 5-1   High-Osmolality Ionic Intravascular Radiopaque Contrast Media—cont'd

	Percentage of iodine
Iothalamate sodium 54.3% (Conray 325)	32.5
Iothalamate sodium 66.8% (Conray 400)	40.0
Iothalamate sodium 80% (Angio Conray)	48.0
COMBINED MEGLUMINE AND SODIUM SALTS	
Diatrizoate meglumine 28.5% Diatrizoate sodium 29.1% (Renovist II)	31.0
Diatrizoate meglumine 34.3% Diatrizoate sodium 35.0% (Renovist)	37.0
Diatrizoate meglumine 50.0% Diatrizoate sodium 25.0% (Hypaque-M 75%)	38.5
Diatrizoate meglumine 52.0% Diatrizoate sodium 8.0% (Angiovist 292) (MD-60) (Renografin-60)	29.3
Diatrizoate meglumine 60.0% Diatrizoate sodium 30.0% (Hypaque-M 90%)	46.2
Diatrizoate meglumine 66.0% Diatrizoate sodium 10.0% (Angiovist 370) (Hypaque-76) (MD-76) (Renografin-76)	37.0
Iothalamate meglumine 52.0% Iothalamate sodium 26.0% (Vascoray)	40.0

Table 5-2 Low-Osmolality Nonionic Intravascular Radiopaque Contrast Media

	Percentage of iodine
Iohexol (Omnipaque)	43.36
Iopamidol 26% (Isovue-128)	12.8
Iopamidol 41% (Isovue-200) (Isovue-M 200)	20.0
Iopamidol 61% (Isovue-300) (Isovue-M 300)	30.0
Iopamidol 76% (Isovue-370)	37.0
Ioversol 34% (Optiray 160)	16.0
Ioversol 51% (Optiray 240)	24.0
Ioversol 68% (Optiray 320)	32.0
Metrizamide (Amipaque)	48.25

Table 5-3 Low-Osmolality Ionic Intravascular Radiopaque Contrast Media

	Percentage of iodine
COMBINED MEGLUMINE AND SODIUM SALTS	
Ioxaglate meglumine 39.3% Ioxaglate sodium 19.6% (Hexabrix)	32.0

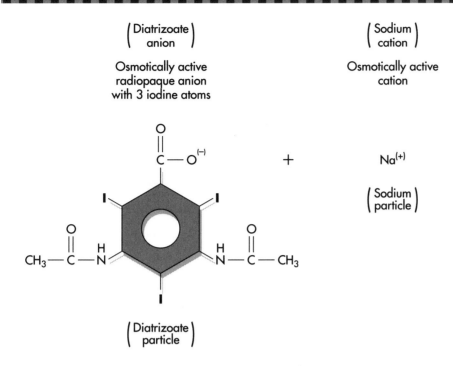

Diatrizoate sodium

Fig. 5-3 Representation of ratio-1.5 ionic ROCM. Diatrizoate sodium contains one osmotically active anion and one osmotically active cation, for a total of two osmotically active particles when in solution. Diatrizoate sodium contains three iodine (I) atoms per every two osmotically active particles to constitute a ratio of 3:2, which equals 1.5.

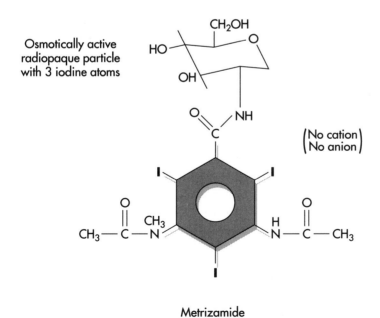

Metrizamide

Fig. 5-4 Representation of ratio-3.0 nonionic ROCM. Metrizamide contains one osmotically active particle when in solution. It does not dissociate into cations and anions. Metrizamide contains three iodine (I) atoms per every osmotically active particle to constitute a ratio of 3:1, which equals 3.0.

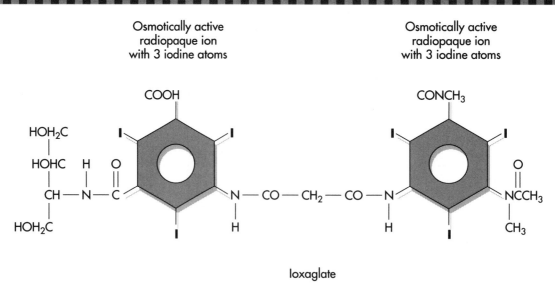

Osmotically active
radiopaque ion
with 3 iodine atoms

Osmotically active
radiopaque ion
with 3 iodine atoms

Ioxaglate

Fig. 5-5   Representation of ratio-3.0 ionic ROCM. Ioxaglate contains two osmotically active ions when in solution. Iotriol contains a total of six iodine atoms per every 2 osmotically active particles to constitute a ratio of 6:2, which equals 3.0.

These are also considered to be ratio-3.0 media because there are six iodine atoms and two dissociated particles per molecule for a ratio of 6:2, which equals 3:1.

Distribution

Intravascular ROCM consist of large molecules, possessing molecular weights ranging between 600 and 1700, with poor lipid (fat) solubility. Consequently, intravascular ROCM do not cross cellular membranes well and are primarily distributed into the bloodstream.

In general, the various intravascular ROCM provide immediate contrast-enhanced visibility to (1) veins and arteries after rapid injection or (2) heart and major thoracic vessels when instilled intravascularly into the heart chambers. Urinary tract visibility is enhanced within 15 minutes of rapid intravenous (IV) injection or within 30 minutes of starting a slow IV infusion in patients with normal renal function; urinary tract visibility may be significantly delayed or not occur at all in patients suffering renal dysfunction or failure. (See Figs. 5-6 and 5-7.)

Tight endothelial junctions forming a blood-brain barrier prevent significant distribution of ROCM into the *normal* central nervous system. A small amount of ROCM may be distributed into the cerebrospinal fluid via the choroid plexus. ROCM will be distributed into and can be used to define brain tumors that lack a blood-brain barrier; pathologic tissues often contain membranes that are less obstructive, thus more permeable, to ROCM. Contrast enhancement of the brain may require up to

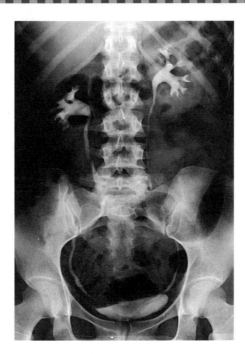

Fig. 5-6 Urogram.

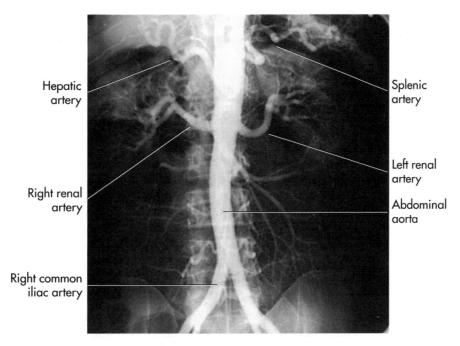

Hepatic
artery

Splenic
artery

Right renal
artery

Left renal
artery

Abdominal
aorta

Right common
iliac artery

Fig. 5-7 Abdominal aortogram.

40 minutes for the ROCM to reach the site; in general, when intravascular ROCM are used to visualize tissue compartments, time is allowed for the ROCM to distribute into them.

Excretion

Intravascular ROCM are excreted primarily via the kidneys; they are concentrated in the kidneys and subsequently opacify the entire renal system. Generally, renal parenchyma is opacified first, followed by the tubular structures, renal calyces, and pelvis, and ending with the ureter and bladder. In normal renal function, up to 100% of an intravascular dose is excreted in 24 hours. A very small percent may be excreted into the intestines via the hepatic-biliary system. Several days may be required for complete excretion in patients suffering renal impairment. Consequently, these patients have much lower to no opacification in the kidneys because up to 50% of the ROCM may be eliminated via the hepatic-biliary system, thus opacifying the biliary and gastrointestinal tracts.

One IV ROCM, iodamide meglumine, is eliminated principally by the hepatic-biliary system and is thus used primarily for cholecystography and cholangiography; this agent has for the most part been replaced by safer methods such as ultrasonography and CT scanning.

ENTERAL RADIOPAQUE CONTRAST MEDIA

Enteral ROCM are used to diagnose and evaluate disorders of the gastrointestinal system. They may also be used to help define the cardiac shadow. Enteral ROCM can be broken down into the categories of aqueous solutions, suspensions, and tablets.

Solutions

Diatrizoate meglumine and **diatrizoate sodium** solutions are used for oral or rectal administration to aid in the diagnosis of gastrointestinal tract disorders. Generally, these solutions are used when barium sulfate suspension is potentially harmful, such as in GI perforation. The high osmolality of these agents causes significant osmotic action within the gastrointestinal tract. This leads to significant dilution of the iodine as well as a profuse diarrhea, systemic hypovolemia, dehydration, and electrolyte imbalance. Iodine dilution leads to less definitive diagnostics; this, along with the adverse effect profile of iodine, is the reason why barium sulfate is often the preferred diagnostic GI agent. The diatrizoate compounds are preferred over barium sulfate for computed tomography, because of less artifact production.

Radiodensity occurs immediately in the esophagus and stomach after oral administration, but may take 15 to 90 minutes for the duodenum. Immediate radiodensity occurs in the rectum and colon following rectal administration.

Gastrointestinal ROCM are not absorbed through the gastrointestinal wall and are thus distributed solely into the GI lumen. These are excreted by the GI tract into the feces.

Suspensions

Barium sulfate is an ROCM suspension that is used for oral or rectal administration to aid in the diagnosis of GI tract disorders. Barium is radiodense in the same manner as iodine. Radiodensity occurs immediately in the esophagus and stomach after oral administration, but may take 15 to 90 minutes for the duodenum. Immediate radiodensity occurs in the rectum and colon following rectal administration. (See Fig. 5-8.)

Barium sulfate is generally the preferred GI ROCM because it provides a more thorough visualization of structures, especially the mucosa, without extensive local adverse effects. Barium sulfate may produce significant artifact in CT evaluation of the GI tract and thus is not the preferred agent for this radiologic exam.

Barium sulfate is not absorbed through the gastrointestinal wall and thus is distributed solely into the GI lumen. It is excreted by the GI tract into the feces.

Tablets

Iocetamic acid (Cholebrine) is an oral ROCM used for opacifying the gallbladder. Absorption varies from person to person, but the gallbladder can generally be visualized approximately 10 to 15 hours after oral administration. (See Fig. 5-9.)

The majority of iocetamic acid is excreted into the urine 48 hours after administration. Some is excreted via the biliary system into the feces.

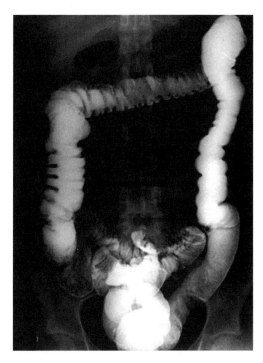

Fig. 5-8 Barium-filled large intestine.

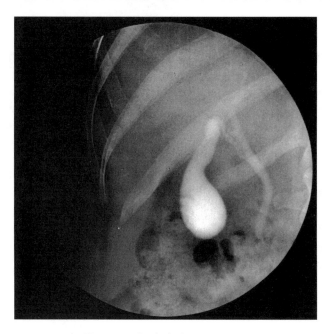

Fig. 5-9 Oral cholecystogram.

CONCLUSION

Radiopaque contrast media are diagnostic agents of high density, most of which contain iodine molecules. The iodine is an integral component in that radiopacity is produced by this molecule. ROCM are divided into various chemical categories and dosage forms.

Learning Exercises

Abbreviations
Spell out the abbreviation below.

1. ROCM:
radiopaque contrast media

True-False
Circle T for true or F for false.

1. T (F) All ROCM used for roentgenography are derivatives of triio-dinated benzoic acid.

2. (T) F Radiopaque contrast media are high-density pharmacologic agents used to visualize low-contrast tissues in the body.

3. T (F) Radiopaque contrast media are not available in enteral form; they are available in parenteral form only.

4. (T) F Ionic ROCM exist in salt form, and nonionic ROCM exist in nonsalt form.

5. (T) F Diatrizoate solutions are used for oral or rectal administration to aid in the diagnosis of gastrointestinal tract disorders.

6. T (F) Barium sulfate is absorbed through the gastrointestinal wall.

7. (T) F Iocetamic acid is an oral ROCM used for opacifying the gall-bladder.

Multiple-Choice Questions
Place a check before the letter of the correct answer.

1. Most radiopaque contrast media used for roentgenography are derivatives of which of the following?
_____ **a.** Barium sulfate
_____ **b.** Triiodinated benzoic acid
_____ **c.** Lead oxide
_____ **d.** Iocetamic acid

2. What is the term for the concentration of osmotically active particles in solution?
_____ **a.** Osmosis
_____ **b.** Osmolality
_____ **c.** Osmotic activity
_____ **d.** Osmolarity

3. What is the term for a negatively charged particle?
   ____ **a.** Electron
   ____ **c.** Anion
   ____ **b.** Cation
   ____ **d.** Proton

4. Why is barium sulfate not used during computed tomography examinations?
   ____ **a.** Danger of electrical shock
   ____ **b.** Creation of image artifacts
   ____ **c.** Nonvisualization of the mucosa
   ____ **d.** Insufficient kilovoltage to penetrate the contrast medium

5. If the kidneys are functioning normally, what percentage of an intravascular ROCM dose is excreted in a 24-hour period?
   ____ **a.** 100%
   ____ **b.** 75%
   ____ **c.** 50%
   ____ **d.** 25%

6. To visualize the gallbladder, ROCM are administered most commonly in which of the following forms?
   ____ **a.** Suspensions
   ____ **b.** Solutions
   ____ **c.** Injections
   ____ **d.** Tablets

7. After injection of an intravascular ROCM, visualization of the kidneys should begin within what period of time?
   ____ **a.** 5 to 10 minutes
   ____ **b.** 15 to 30 minutes
   ____ **c.** 30 to 45 minutes
   ____ **d.** 1 hour

Fill-in-the-Blank Questions

1. A ___neg.___ charged particle is known as an anion, and a ___pos-___ charged particle is known as a cation.

2. A ___osmotic agent___ will attract water so that a dilutional effect can occur to equilibrate pressures between two permeable or semipermeable membranes.

3. ___↑___ density of the ROCM alters the attenuation of x-rays, thus enhancing the anatomic image on the radiographic film.

4. ___Iodine___ is an integral component of ROCM because radiopacity is produced by this element.

5. _intravascular_ ROCM are excreted primarily via the kidneys and are concentrated in the kidneys.

6. _intravascular_ ROCM consist of large molecules, with molecular weights ranging from 600 to 1700 and with poor lipid solubility.

Review Questions

1. What is the difference between ratio-1.5 media and ratio-3.0 media?

The ratio of iodine atoms to osmotic actively particles is 3:2 in a ratio 1.5 media and 3:1 in a 3.0 media.

2. Why is iodine used so extensively in ROCM?

B/c it absorbs x-ray photons, thus enhancing contrast.

3. Why do intravascular ROCM tend to remain in the bloodstream?

Large molecules that can not cross cell membranes.

4. Why is iodamide meglumine used primarily for cholecystography and cholangiography?

Auretied by the hepatobiliary system.

5. What are the three broad categories of intravascular ROCM?

highly osmolality ionic ROCM
low osmolality non-ionic ROCM
ionic ROCM

6. When are diatrizoate solutions most commonly used?

when a BaSO4 ~~suspension~~ suspension is potentially harmful such as in GI perforation, or when CT is being used b/c of less artifact production.

6

Pharmacodynamics of Radiopaque Contrast Media

OBJECTIVES

At the conclusion of this chapter you should be able to:
1. List the diagnostic pharmacodynamic effects of radiopaque contrast media.
2. Describe the adverse pharmacodynamic effects of radiopaque contrast media.
3. Discuss examples of screening methods used to evaluate patients prior to introduction of radiopaque contrast media.
4. Identify specific drug-drug interactions with radiopaque contrast media that can cause adverse effects.

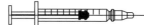

IODINATED RADIOPAQUE CONTRAST MEDIA

Pharmacodynamics, as outlined in Chapter 4, is the study of the actions or outcome elicited by drugs when the site of action is reached. Pharmacodynamic effects can be therapeutic, diagnostic, or adverse. Diagnostic effects of intravascular radiopaque contrast media are a function of the iodine contained within them. Adverse effects elicited by ROCM depend at least partially upon their serum or tissue iodine concentration and osmolality and their calcium-chelating, anticoagulant, and immune system–stimulating abilities.

DIAGNOSTIC PHARMACODYNAMICS

Serum iodine concentration must be within the range of 280 mg/ml to 370 mg/ml for a normal x-ray to reflect the vascular lumen. To achieve this high iodine concentration, the ROCM must contain a large proportion of iodine (see Chapter 5 for iodine concentrations) and be injected intravascularly at a rate equal to or greater than blood flow. If the ROCM is injected slowly, the cardiovascular system will significantly dilute the iodine concentration prior to filming. Rapid intravascular injection thus helps to limit the early dilutional effects that the cardiovascular system has on the iodine. High concentrations of iodine pharmacodynamically prevent the penetration of photons so that a shadow is projected onto the radiographic film.

 For computerized tomography (CT) or digital subtraction angiography (DSA), the serum iodine concentration needs only to be between 2 mg/ml and 8 mg/ml. Thus, either a less concentrated iodine ROCM or a slower intravascular infusion will produce adequate pharmacodynamic action for these imaging procedures.

ADVERSE PHARMACODYNAMICS

Serious adverse effects from ROCM do occur. An estimated one of every 20,000 to 40,000 patients receiving ROCM dies as a result of these effects. Although the odds of death appear low, they become very real if it happens to you or your patient. Thus it is paramount that the technologist understand adverse effects so that proper actions can be instituted as rapidly as possible.

Osmolality Effects

As discussed in Chapter 5, the intravascular ROCM contain a higher osmolar weight than the normal bloodstream. Various physiologic effects are elicited by intravascular administration of high-osmolality ROCM. Intravascular administration of ROCM will cause a transient rise in intravascular osmotic pressure. Fluid from surrounding tissues is then drawn into the vascular lumen to dilute the osmotically active particles. This occurs to equalize pressure between intravascular and extravascular spaces (see Fig. 5-2). These osmotic forces or effects will cause fluid extraction from red blood cells (RBCs), endothelium, and extravascular space.

When fluid is extracted from the RBCs, they shrink and become less pliable. Endothelium water loss also results in endothelial shrinking. The movement of tissue water into the intravascular space as a result of osmotic forces causes short-term extravascular fluid decreases with resultant increased intravascular contents. In other words, there is less fluid outside the vessels and more fluid inside the vessels. This action is thought to be responsible for vasodilation and flushing experienced by most patients receiving intravascular ROCM.

Shortly after injection, the cardiovascular system circulates and dilutes the hyperosmolar ROCM, washing it downstream, eventually producing an intravascular *hypo*osmolar state in comparison to the extravascular space. In other words, the extra particles inside the vessels are moved away in the current of the blood supply, as in a river. When that happens, the fluid on the outside of the vessels no longer needs to dilute the fluid on the inside of the vessels. The extravascular space becomes hyperosmolar because of dehydration, resulting in yet another fluid shift from the intravascular space back to the extravascular or tissue space. This continues until an osmolar equilibrium is reached between intravascular and extravascular spaces. These intravascular-extravascular osmotic shifts produced by the ROCM may be partially responsible for adverse renal effects induced by these agents. Initial increases in renal vessel fluid volume, caused by hyperosmolar fluid shifts, are followed by a prolonged decrease in renal blood flow, which ultimately leads to tissue ischemia (decreased oxygen) with resultant damage. In addition, the urine becomes hyperosmolar when the ROCM is excreted

DID YOU KNOW?

Contrast agents used in magnetic resonance imaging are usually paramagnetic agents designed to enhance the T1 and T2 relaxation times of hydrogen nuclei. These agents have been developed for intravenous, oral, and inhalation administration. Most are introduced intravenously. Gadolinium +3 (Gd^{+3}), which has seven unpaired electrons, has the strongest relaxation rate properties and has proven effective in demonstrating various types of lesions. Because of its high toxicity, it is administered in a complex with DTPA (diethylenetriaminepentaacetic acid) (GD-DTPA) to ensure detoxification.

into it; this will cause an osmotic diuresis, which can result in dehydration of the patient.

Hyperosmolar ROCM injection into the carotid arteries results in intraarterial osmotic pressure changes significant enough to stimulate **baroreceptors** and **chemoreceptors** located at the bifurcation of the aortic arch and carotid arteries. These receptors cause the autonomic nervous system to slow the heart rate down (bradycardia) and produce a drop in aortic pressure. If this occurs, the patient may faint or lose consciousness. This type of reaction has been referred to as a **vasovagal reaction** (Fig. 6-1, *A*); the vagus nerve is stimulated by transient vascular hypertension. When a vasovagal event occurs, the patient becomes symptomatically hypotensive as a result of moderate to severe bradycardia produced by vagus nerve stimulation.

Intravascular osmotic fluid shifts can also result in acute heart failure in patients who already suffer from chronic congestive heart failure (Fig. 6-1, *B*). Signs and symptoms of acute-on-chronic heart failure (acute heart failure superimposed on chronic heart failure) generally include respiratory difficulty with pulmonary edema and may include tachycardia or bradycardia, hypertension or hypotension, cardiac dysrhythmias, cardiorespiratory arrest, and death.

A failing heart has trouble pumping all of the fluid that is presented to it. When osmotic shifts of fluid occur intravascularly, the heart is presented with an increased load, or burden, to pump. The cardiac output then drops as the heart continues to fail. Baroreceptors located in the aortic arch and carotid arteries then send signals to the central nervous system that ultimately cause the release of counterregulatory hormones such as vasopressin, adrenaline, renin, angiotensin I, angiotensin II, and aldosterone. These hormones act to increase the blood pressure by causing fluid retention and vasoconstriction; the goal of the body is to preserve brain function in a state of perceived decreased blood pressure and nutrient (oxygen) supply. Unfortunately, this cycle becomes detrimental to outcome because the heart is already burdened. Vasoconstriction will increase the force against which the heart has to pump, thus causing the heart to work harder and fail quicker. The fluid retention causes an increased volume presenting to the heart for circulation, thus leading to a greater load of fluid, which is a burden to a failing heart. In these cases, it is therapeutic to use diuretics, such as furosemide, to excrete fluid from the body, and cardiac stimulators, such as dobutamine, to increase the strength of the heart. Fig. 6-1,*B*, briefly outlines this effect.

Chelation Effects

ROCM can **chelate** (bind to) calcium ions in the cardiovascular system following injection. Calcium chelation may be one pharmacodynamic mechanism by which adverse heart rhythms such as **electromechanical dissociation (EMD),** cardiac arrest, and sudden death occur in a minority of patients receiving intravascular ROCM. EMD is a heart rhythm disturbance characterized by electrical impulses without cardiac contraction. In other words, the heart monitor shows electrical activity, but the heart is not pumping. A cardiac arrest means simply that the heart ceases

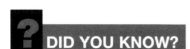

DID YOU KNOW?

Contrast agents are being experimented with for use in sonography using microaggregated albumin. Albumin resembles air bubbles and is being used especially in the determination of fallopian tube patency and during echocardiography.

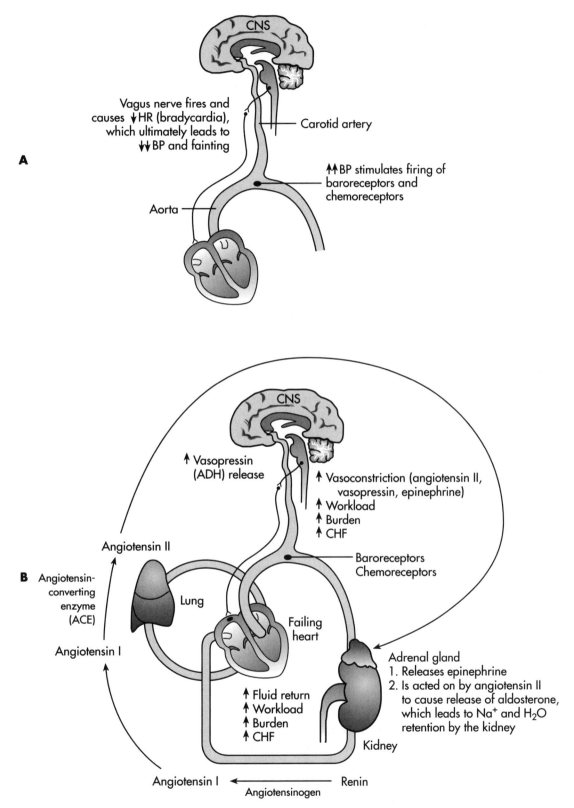

CNS

Vagus nerve fires and
causes ↓HR (bradycardia),
which ultimately leads to
↓↓BP and fainting

A

Carotid artery

↑↑BP stimulates firing of
baroreceptors and
chemoreceptors

Aorta

CNS

↑Vasopressin
(ADH) release

↑Vasoconstriction (angiotensin II,
vasopressin, epinephrine)
↑Workload
↑Burden
↑CHF

Angiotensin II

B Angiotensin-
converting
enzyme
(ACE)

Lung

Angiotensin I

Failing
heart

Baroreceptors
Chemoreceptors

Adrenal gland
1. Releases epinephrine
2. Is acted on by angiotensin II
   to cause release of aldosterone,
   which leads to Na⁺ and H₂O
   retention by the kidney

↑Fluid return
↑Workload
↑Burden
↑CHF

Kidney

Angiotensin I ← Renin
Angiotensinogen

Fig. 6-1   **A,** Vasovagal reaction. **B,** Congestive heart failure with osmotic load added.

to effectively pump blood to maintain life. Sudden death is usually the result of a heart rhythm (ventricular tachycardia and/or fibrillation) that cannot sustain life.

Anticoagulation Effects

High-osmolality ROCM can cause some **anticoagulation** (blood thinning) to occur. This can theoretically result in bleeding and bruising episodes. Low-osmolality ROCM do not appear to produce anticoagulant effects.

Immune System–Like Effects

The immune system is highly complex and consists of various components, including physical barriers such as the skin, gastric acid, duodenal alkali, and respiratory cilia and biochemical defenses such as inflammation, lysosymes, complement proteins, and immunoglobulins. It is the biochemical defenses that are thought to have a role in the immediately life-threatening reaction mimicking an anaphylactic reaction that can occur with ROCM. Important to note is that this reaction is not absolutely characterized as anaphylaxis, but more appropriately is *anaphylactoid* in nature. To understand this distinction, we must first understand what true anaphylaxis entails.

Anaphylaxis is an immediately life-threatening systemic hypersensitivity reaction. Patients suffering anaphylaxis may exhibit any combination of nausea, vomiting, diarrhea, hives, rash, flushing, cyanosis, pallor, lightheadedness, unconsciousness, seizures, stridor, wheezing, respiratory distress, bronchospasm, laryngeal edema, cardiac dysrhythmias, marked hypotension, vascular collapse, and cardiorespiratory arrest. Anaphylaxis is often fatal if treatment is not immediate. Within minutes of exposure to a foreign substance, acting as an antigen, a complex forms with an endogenous antibody known as immunoglobulin E (IgE) and located on a mast cell.

Mast cells are connective tissue cells that contain the chemicals histamine, leukotriene (also known as "slow-reacting substance of anaphylaxis" [SRS-A]), eosinophil chemotactic factor, neutrophil chemotactic factor, kininogenase, arylsulfatase A, exglycosides, prostaglandin, thromboxane, platelet-activating factor, monohydroxyeicosatetraenoic acid (HETE), and hydroperoxyeicosatetraenoic acid (HPETE). Mast cells are located in skin, synovium, and mesentery, around large and small blood vessels, in the mucosa of the respiratory tract, and in the subserosal and submucosal layers of the gastrointestinal tract.

Anaphylaxis is generally referred to as a type I hypersensitivity reaction, which requires a first-time exposure to the antigen (i.e., the foreign substance) at some time in the patient's history. The first exposure results in the substance forming an **antigen-antibody complex** that "sensitizes" the mast cells to future events (Fig. 6-2, *A*). An immediate reaction does not occur at this point. It is the second exposure to the same substance that causes IgE to stimulate the "sensitized" mast cell to release its dangerous chemicals. In combination, these chemicals cause the life-threatening effects described earlier. This type of reaction is com-

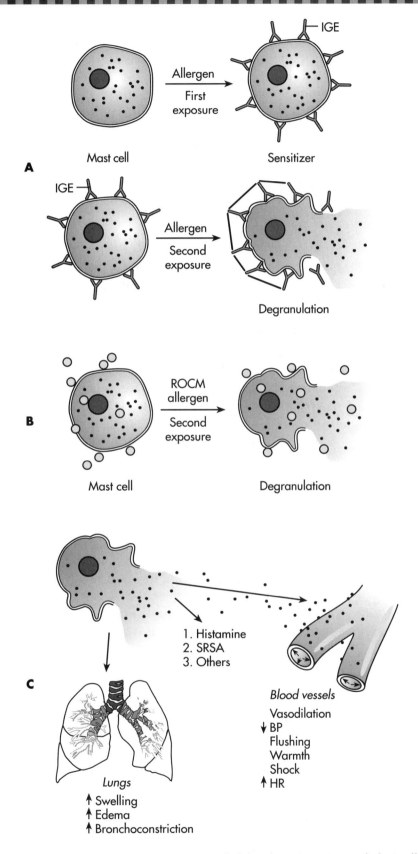

Fig. 6-2 **A,** Anaphylactic reaction. **B,** Anaphylactoid reaction. **C,** Anaphylaxis effects.

mon in patients who are allergic to bee stings; the first sting poses no threat, but weeks or years later a second sting may be fatal.

Radiopaque contrast media may cause what is termed anaphylactoid reactions (Fig. 6-2, *B*). This type of reaction clinically mimics the anaphylactic reaction, but no prior exposure to ROCM is necessary to "sensitize" the mast cell. Upon first exposure to the ROCM, mast cells may release their chemicals to cause an anaphylaxis-like, or anaphylactoid, adverse effect. Therefore, a history of previous exposure is not relevant to the possibility of anaphylactoid reaction. This reaction is just as lethal as anaphylaxis (Fig. 6-2, *C*). For this reason a medical imaging technologist needs a functional understanding of emergency procedures.

The biochemical pathways for anaphylactoid reactions are not well known at this time. Up to 40% of patients who have suffered an anaphylactoid event as a result of ROCM in the past may suffer one again. However, it is controversial whether to administer prophylactic medications such as antihistamines and corticosteroids to such patients.

Renal Dysfunction

Radiopaque contrast media are responsible for approximately 10% of all **acute renal failure (ARF)** events and are the third most common cause of hospital-acquired ARF. Reported incidences are 2% following angiography, 2% to 25% following intravenous pyelography, and 50% to 100% in patients who suffer from renal nephropathy caused by diabetes.

Patients who suffer ROCM ARF generally present with a mild, reversible, nonoliguric (i.e., urine output is greater than 400 ml/day) event of short duration. The serum creatinine concentration (a renal function test) begins to rise in the first 24 hours following intravenous ROCM, peaks in 2 to 4 days, and normalizes in 7 to 10 days.

Oliguric ARF does occur in some patients. If this is the case, urine output does not exceed 400 ml/day. In such cases, the renal failure may not be reversible and the serum creatinine does not normalize.

The pharmacodynamic mechanisms for ROCM-induced ARF are theorized to include direct renal tubular toxicity, renal ischemia due to the osmotic fluid shifts discussed earlier, intratubular obstruction from precipitated proteins and/or uric acid/calcium oxalate crystals, and, least likely, immunologic factors.

Patients at risk for ARF following intravenous ROCM are those with preexisting renal compromise, diabetes with concomitant renal dysfunction, or possibly dehydration.

Diabetes alone was historically considered a high risk, but now is considered one only if concomitant renal dysfunction exists. Diabetic patients with serum creatinine levels greater than 4.5 mg/dl have been reported to suffer a 100% incidence of ARF following ROCM. Dehydration prior to ROCM injection is not a major risk factor, provided the patient is hydrated following the exam. (Dehydration alone can result in significant ARF if not treated.)

Thyroid Storm

A rare but potentially fatal adverse pharmacodynamic effect that has occurred following the administration of iodine-rich ROCM is **thyroid storm.** This generally occurs in patients who suffer **decompensated thyrotoxicosis.** Decompensated thyrotoxicosis is a condition in which the body becomes unable to tolerate thyroid hormones. In these patients, the iodine from the ROCM can cause the thyroid to either produce or liberate amounts of thyroid hormone that exceed the body's tolerance level; important to note is that this does not imply that the serum thyroid hormone levels are in excess of normal values, but rather that they are in excess of the patient's ability to tolerate them.

Signs and symptoms of thyroid storm include fever, tachycardia (rapid heart rate), diaphoresis (sweating), agitation, nervousness, and emotional instability. Untreated, thyroid storm can lead to congestive heart failure, refractory pulmonary edema, cardiovascular collapse, coma, and death within 24 hours.

As an imaging professional, it may not be your responsibility to diagnose this disorder, but you can always help refresh the memory of those with whom the responsibility lies. Please keep in mind that thyroid storm can have a fatal outcome!

GENERAL ADVERSE REACTIONS

General adverse effects that may or may not be related to any of the adverse effects mentioned so far include nausea, vomiting, flushing with a generalized feeling of warmth, rhinitis, lacrimation, sneezing, itching, rash, angioedema, generalized edema, cramps, excessive salivation, salivary gland swelling, diaphoresis, retching and choking, metallic taste in mouth, decreased white blood cells, chills, fever, and disseminated intravascular coagulation.

Adverse central nervous system effects may include nervousness, confusion, anxiety, headaches, dizziness, tremors, agitation, and seizures. At the site of injection the patient may suffer thrombophlebitis, pain, burning, stinging, numbness, bruising, necrosis, and sloughing of tissue (if extravasation occurs).

ROCM can lead to sickling of red blood cells as a result of osmotic fluid shifts in patients who suffer sickle cell anemia, ARF in patients suffering multiple myeloma (cancer of serum proteins), hypertensive crisis in patients suffering pheochromocytoma (adrenal gland tumor that releases large amounts of adrenaline), and intractable seizures in patients suffering subarachnoid hemorrhage.

ROCM do cross placental barriers and should not be used in pregnant women unless benefits far exceed risks.

SCREENING

In light of all the serious adverse effects that can occur by injection of intravascular ROCM, the imaging technologist should use a screening method that includes the assessment of patient medical history and current renal function status. Questions that should be answered prior to administering intravascular ROCM include at least those listed in the box on p. 76.

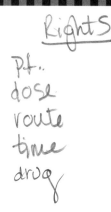

Rights
Pt.
dose
route
time
drug

? DID YOU KNOW?

Dr. Werner Forssman was experimenting with cardiac catheterization techniques in the late 1930s. Finding no willing human subjects, he cut down to his own brachial artery no fewer than nine separate times and introduced a urinary catheter into his own heart. The medical community thought he was insane and banned him from all teaching and medical appointments. In 1956 he was awarded the Nobel Prize.

QUESTIONS TO BE ANSWERED
BEFORE ADMINISTRATION OF ROCM

1. History of allergies to medications?
2. History of intolerance to iodine?
3. History of adverse reactions to radiopaque contrast media?
4. History of asthma or breathing difficulties?
5. History of cardiac disease?
   a. Congestive failure
   b. Cardiac dysrhythmias
   c. Hypertension
   d. Hypotension
6. History of renal disease?
   a. Chronic renal failure
   b. Acute renal failure
   c. Current blood urea nitrogen (BUN) concentration (a renal function test)
   d. Current serum creatinine concentration (a renal function test)
7. Current medications?
8. History of diabetes?
9. History of sickle cell anemia (in black patients)?
10. History of multiple myeloma?
11. Is the patient pregnant (females only)?
12. Current central nervous system trauma?

DRUG-DRUG INTERACTIONS

Many patients requiring intravascular ROCM administration have an indwelling intravenous catheter through which other medications are to be infused. Occasionally, an intravenous drug may be required to improve visualization in a vascular bed or to counteract severe adverse effects that may occur as a result of ROCM. For instance, vasodilators are used to improve delivery of ROCM to small arteries that may be inaccessible otherwise. Vasoconstrictors are administered to decrease delivery of ROCM to normal vascular beds in order to help visualize vascular beds that are not normal and are supplying a tumor. Vascular beds within a tumor may not respond to vasoconstrictors, as normal vessels do, because they lack elasticity and receptor density; therefore, ROCM will be specifically delivered to the tumor vessels when vasoconstrictors are used. These adjunct medications are generally injected immediately prior to ROCM injection. Drug-drug interactions in the form of chemical incompatibilities may occur between ROCM and these adjunct drugs.

Chemical incompatibilities that produce insoluble precipitates can theoretically lead to occlusion of intravenous catheters and/or possibly a chemically induced embolism that can occlude small vessels in its path. The severity can range from mild to death, depending on which vessel the occlusion occurs in. Thus it is paramount that the technologist understand which drug-ROCM combinations are known to cause this phenomenon and how to circumvent the problem.

Diatrizoate meglumine, diatrizoate sodium, ioxaglate, and iothalamate are the more active ROCM with regard to forming precipitates with other intravenous drugs. (See Table 6-1.) Iopamidol and iohexol have not been found to chemically interact with the medications listed in Table 6-1. Other medications tested and found to cause no precipitate with the above ROCM include prostaglandin E_1, nitroglycerin, vasopressin, epinephrine hydrochloride, pheniramine maleate, benzylpenicillin sodium, ampicillin sodium, chloramphenicol sodium succinate, lidocaine hydrochloride, heparin sodium, urokinase, and hydrocortisone sodium succinate.

If two incompatible drugs must be administered to a patient, it is recommended that physiologic saline (0.9% sodium chloride) be used to flush the intravenous catheter prior to each drug. If the chemical compatibility between two drugs is not known, it is prudent to assume that they are incompatible and administer a physiologic saline flush between doses. In any case, it is probably safest to flush the intravenous line between doses of two drugs, regardless of known compatibility data.

Other drug-drug interactions that many fear include the possibility of an increase in seizure activity when phenothiazine antinauseants are used following intrathecal administration of ROCM. Also, the use of ROCM in patients who take antihypertensive medications may lead to prolonged and exaggerated hypotensive effects.

BARIUM SULFATE

Enteral barium sulfate can cause both gastrointestinal and respiratory adverse effects. In the GI tract, barium sulfate produces an insoluble pre-

Table 6-1 ROCM and Common Intravenous Drugs Forming Precipitates

The following radiopaque contrast media, when mixed with any of the listed intravenous drugs, may form precipitates that may occlude intravenous catheters or produce chemically induced emboli.

Diatrizoate meglumine +	Papaverine hydrochloride (smooth muscle relaxant)
	Phentolamine mesylate (antiadrenergic)
	Diphenhydramine hydrochloride (antihistimine)
	Cimetidine hydrochloride (stomach antacid)
	Diazepam (sedative and tranquilizer)
	Meperidine hydrochloride (narcotic analgesic)
	Protamine sulfate (heparin antagonist)
Diatrizoate sodium +	Papaverine hydrochloride
	Phentolamine mesylate
	Diphenhydramine hydrochloride
	Meperidine hydrochloride
	Protamine sulfate
Ioxaglate +	Tolazoline hydrochloride (peripheral vasodilator)
	Gentamicin sulfate (aminoglycoside antibiotic)
	Papaverine hydrochloride
	Phentolamine mesylate
	Diphenhydramine hydrochloride
	Cimetidine hydrochloride
	Protamine sulfate
Iothalamate +	Phentolamine mesylate

cipitate with calcium to form barium fecaliths, which can lead to constipation, intestinal obstruction, ulceration, and/or perforation as a result of impaction of the colon. Surgical intervention may be required to remove them. Distention, cramping, and diarrhea may also occur. Rarely, chemically induced appendicitis has occurred in patients who retain barium in the appendix. If intestinal perforation occurs, large amounts of barium can cause intestinal infarction, desiccation, severe peritonitis, and death.

Aspiration of barium sulfate into the lungs generally does not cause harm, provided the amount aspirated is small. Large aspirates may lead to pneumonitis and nodular granulomas of both lung tissue and lymph nodes. Asphyxiation and death have been reported in at least one case of barium sulfate aspiration.

CONCLUSION

Radiopaque contrast media have various pharmacodynamic actions that are important for the imaging technologist to comprehend. Diagnostic effects rely on adequate ROCM concentrations at the site. Adverse effects and drug-drug interactions suffered from ROCM are generally mild, but can be very life-threatening. The competent imaging professional will strive to understand such reactions.

Learning Exercises

Abbreviations

Spell out each of the abbreviations below.

1. DSA:

digital subtraction angiography

2. EMD:

electromechanical dissociation

3. ARF:

acute renal failure

True-False

Circle T for true or F for false.

1. T (**F**) Low-osmolality radiopaque contrast media can cause anticoagulation to occur.

2. (**T**) F Radiopaque contrast media do cross placental barriers.

3. T (**F**) Intravascular administration of ROCM will cause a transient decrease in intravascular osmotic pressure.

4. (**T**) F Sometimes ROCM do cause serious adverse effects.

5. T (**F**) When a vasovagal event occurs, the patient becomes symptomatically hypertensive as a result of moderate to severe bradycardia.

6. (**T**) F Calcium chelation may be one pharmocodynamic mechanism by which adverse heart rhythms, cardiac arrest, and sudden death occur in a minority of patients receiving intravascular ROCM.

7. (**T**) F High-osmolality ROCM can cause some anticoagulation that can result in bleeding and bruising.

8. T (**F**) Even without immediate treatment, anaphylaxis is not often fatal.

9. (**T**) F Decompensated thyrotoxicosis is a condition in which the body becomes unable to tolerate thyroid hormones.

10. **T** **F** ROCM are responsible for approximately 10% of all acute renal failure events and are the third most common cause of hospital-acquired acute renal failure.

Multiple-Choice Questions

Place a check before the letter of the correct answer.

1. In order to visualize the vascular lumen via normal x-ray exposure, the blood iodine concentration must be within which of the following ranges?
   _____ **a.** 150 to 200 mg/ml
   _____ **b.** 220 to 260 mg/ml
   _____ **c.** 280 to 370 mg/ml
   _____ **d.** 400 to 480 mg/ml

2. What is the term for a heart rhythm disturbance characterized by electrical impulses without cardiac contraction?
   _____ **a.** Electromechanical dissociation
   _____ **b.** Chelation
   _____ **c.** Tachycardia
   _____ **d.** Fibrillation

3. What is the term for an immediately life-threatening systemic hypersensitivity reaction?
   _____ **a.** Tachycardia
   _____ **b.** Stridor
   _____ **c.** Anaphylaxis
   _____ **d.** Hypotension

4. Radiopaque contrast media are responsible for approximately what percentage of all acute renal failure events?
   _____ **a.** 5%
   _____ **b.** 10%
   _____ **c.** 50%
   _____ **d.** 75%

5. In oliguric acute renal failure, urine output does not exceed what amount?
   _____ **a.** 100 ml/day
   _____ **b.** 200 ml/day
   _____ **c.** 300 ml/day
   _____ **d.** 400 ml/day

6. When a patient is assessed prior to introduction of a radiopaque contrast medium, it is vitally important to evaluate the medical history and which of the following?

_____ **a.** Current renal function status

_____ **b.** Mode of medium introduction

_____ **c.** Injection site

_____ **d.** Subsequent diagnostic tests

7. Thyroid storm generally occurs in patients who suffer which of the following?

_____ **a.** Tachycardia

_____ **b.** Decompensated thyrotoxicosis

_____ **c.** Hypothyroidism

_____ **d.** Congestive heart failure

8. What is the percentage of ARF incidents following angiography?

_____ **a.** 1%

_____ **b.** 2%

_____ **c.** 10%

_____ **d.** 25%

9. The pharmacodynamic mechanisms for ROCM-induced ARF are theorized to include which of the following?

_____ **a.** Direct renal tubular toxicity

_____ **b.** Renal ischemia

_____ **c.** Intratubular obstruction

_____ **d.** All of the above

10. Which of the following can result from large amounts of barium sulfate being aspirated?

_____ **a.** Death

_____ **b.** Pneumonitis

_____ **c.** Granulomas of lung tissue and lymph nodes

_____ **d.** All of the above

Fill-in-the-Blank Questions

1. An immediately life-threatening systemic hypersensitivity reaction is known as _anaphylaxis_.

2. A _chemoreceptor_ is a sensory nerve cell activated by chemical stimuli.

3. ROCM can lead to sickling of red blood cells as a result of osmotic fluid shifts in patients who suffer from _sickle cell anemia_

4. ROCM cross _placenta barriers_ and should not be used in pregnant women unless benefits far exceed risks.

5. Patients at risk for _ARF_ following intravascular ROCM administration include those with preexisting renal compromise, diabetes with concomitant renal dysfunction, or dehydration.

6. Signs and symptoms of _thyroid storm_ include fever, tachycardia, diaphoresis, agitation, nervousness, and emotional instability.

7. Because of the serious effects that can occur by injection of intravascular ROCM, the imaging technologist should use a screening method that includes _assessment of patient medical history_ and _current renal functional status_.

8. _Vasodilators_ are used to improve delivery of ROCM to small arteries that may be inaccessible otherwise.

Review Questions

1. Why is a history of previous exposure to a drug or ROCM not enough to predict the possibility of a hypersensitivity reaction?

   Mast cells may respond to the first exposure w/ anaphylaxis.

2. What should be done to ensure safe administration of two or more incompatible drugs? What should be done if information on drug-drug compatibility is not available?

   Assume incompatibility & flush line w/ saline to prevent drug - drug contact.

Routes of Drug Administration

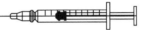

7

OBJECTIVES

At the conclusion of this chapter you should be able to:

1. List and define the "five rights" of drug administration.
2. Cite the advantages and disadvantages of the various routes of medication administration.
3. Identify the landmarks for the administration of medications via the intramuscular route.
4. Identify specific procedures used to maintain patient safety during the preparation and administration of medications.
5. Recognize common abbreviations and symbols related to medication administration.

INTRODUCTION

Prior to giving a patient any medication (drug), the medical imaging technologist should always adhere to the *five rights* of drug administration.

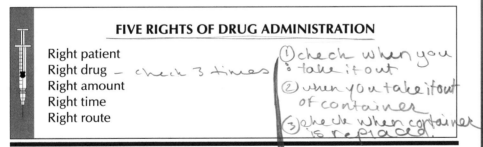

FIVE RIGHTS OF DRUG ADMINISTRATION

Right patient
Right drug — check 3 times
Right amount
Right time
Right route

(handwritten annotations:) ① check when you take it out ② when you take it out of container ③ check when container is replaced.

The following commonsense reminders can help ensure that the *right patient* receives the *right drug* in the *right amount* at the *right time* via the *right route. Check the drug name carefully* by always reading the label on the container three times: once when the container is removed from the shelf, again when the drug is removed from the container, and a third time when the container is replaced. Since it is now common for drug companies to prepare contrast in "prefilled" syringes, be sure to check the name on the prefilled syringe as it is taken from the package to ensure that it matches the name on the outside of the package. Also, remember that the names of different drugs may sound similar (e.g., Renografin vs. Gastrografin). Never use a drug that is unlabeled or expired. Always check the label for the drug's expiration date. Under no circumstances should an expired drug be used. To prevent error, it is good practice never to administer a drug someone else has prepared. If you must prepare a drug for another health professional to administer, always show the container to the individual who will administer the drug before you hand him or her the medication. If an error is made, *everyone* involved is responsible! Make sure you have done everything *right* for your patient.

Dose measurement must be done carefully and accurately to ensure that the *right amount* is used. Inaccurate measurements can lead to significant toxicity. When you are preparing to administer an injectable drug, it is also important to select the right size and type of syringe and needle. Some medication may require a large-bore needle because of medication viscosity or the need for rapid injection.

Check the patient's arm band for proper identification and ask for his or her name to ensure that you are administering the drug to the *right patient.* If the arm band does not coincide with the name given, do not administer the drug. If the patient does not state his or her name as written on the arm band, do not administer the drug. Keep in mind that confused patients may answer to any name given. Make the patient verbalize his or her name prior to your stating the name. If he or she is too young to speak or is unable to speak, ask a parent or someone present to identify the patient. Last, address the patient by name before administering the drug.

The *right time* for administering a drug is usually indicated by the physician or practitioner responsible for ordering the drug. As a general rule, the medical imaging technologist does not determine the time but should administer the drug at the time specified.

The physician usually specifies the route by which the drug should be administered. The technologist must be familiar with medical terminology to ensure that the drug is administered by the *right route.*

Drugs may be administered via the oral, sublingual, topical, rectal, and parenteral routes. General principles associated with each route of administration will be discussed.

ORAL ROUTE

The **oral** route is the most common method of drug administration. Oral administration is the safest, most economical, and most convenient way of giving medication. Therefore, it is the preferred route unless some distinct advantage is to be gained by using another route or a contraindication to oral administration is present. Most drugs undergo absorption in the small intestine; few are absorbed in the stomach and colon. This process is further explained in Chapter 3. Drug effects are generally *slower* and *less efficient* when a drug is given orally rather than parenterally. When receiving drugs by the oral route, the patient must be conscious and the head should be elevated to aid in swallowing.

A major advantage of the oral route is that it allows for the easiest retrieval of a drug in overdose situations. Until a drug is dissolved and absorbed, it may be retrieved by lavage/catharsis or may be adsorbed to block absorption. The parenteral route does not allow for this.

Disadvantages of oral administration of certain drugs are that (1) they may have an objectionable odor or taste or be bulky to swallow, (2) they may harm or discolor the teeth, (3) they may irritate the gastric mucosa, causing nausea and vomiting, (4) they may be aspirated by a seriously ill or uncooperative individual, (5) they may be destroyed by digestive enzymes, and (6) they may be inappropriate for some patients, such as those who must be given nothing by mouth.

SUBLINGUAL AND BUCCAL ROUTES

Sublingual administration is performed by placing the drug under the tongue for disolution and absorption. The thin epithelium and network of capillaries on the underside of the tongue permit drug absorption. Drugs administered via this route will gain access to the general circulation without traversing the liver or being affected by gastric and intestinal enzymes. Thus, the drug potency may be enhanced. This also applies to **buccal** administration, in which a tablet is held in the mouth in the pocket between gums and cheek for local dissolution and absorption. Nitroglycerin tablets and morphine sulfate solution are two examples of drugs commonly administered via the sublingual and buccal routes.

The number of drugs that can be given sublingually or buccally is limited (e.g., nitroglycerin tablets). The drug must dissolve readily, and the patient must be able to cooperate. The patient must understand that the drug is not to be swallowed and that taking a drink must be avoided until the drug has been absorbed. However, usually little harm is done if a sublingual drug is inadvertently swallowed. *Note:* It is unclear, in some cases, whether a drug is absorbed under the tongue or actually swallowed and absorbed in the intestinal tract.

TOPICAL ROUTE

The **topical** route of drug administration involves the application of a drug directly onto the skin or mucous membrane. The drug is diffused through the skin or membrane and absorbed into the bloodstream. These medications are applied for the following effects:

1. **Astringent:** resulting in vasoconstriction, tissue contraction, and decreased secretions and sensitivity, thereby counteracting inflammatory effects
2. **Antiseptic** or **bacteriostatic:** to inhibit growth and development of microorganisms (e.g., Betadine or Bactroban)
3. **Emollient:** for a soothing and softening effect to overcome dryness and hardness (e.g., lanolin)
4. Cleansing: for the removal of dirt, debris, secretions, or crusts (e.g., Hibiclens)
5. **Anesthetic:** to remove the sensation of pain (e.g., benzocaine)
6. **Antihistamine:** for manifestations due to allergic reactions (e.g., Benadryl cream)

Topical medications may be applied in the form of a lotion, tincture (alcoholic solution), ointment or cream, foam, spray, gel, wet dressing, tam-

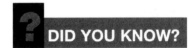

DID YOU KNOW?

In the United States, the elderly hospitalized patient is prescribed an average of 9.1 drugs per day. In Canada, 7.1 drugs are prescribed daily, while Israel follows with 6.3 per day, New Zealand with 5.8 per day and Scotland with 4.6 per day.

pon, bath, or soak. The effectiveness of medicinals applied to the skin for local effect is limited by the fact that highly specialized layers of skin resist penetration of many (not all) foreign substances to protect the internal body environment. Topical absorption is increased when the skin is thin or macerated, when there is increased drug concentration, when there is prolonged contact of the drug with the skin, or when the drug is combined with a solvent-penetrant. The mucous membranes absorb drugs much more readily because they are not **keratinized.** Keratin is a scleroprotein that is the principal constituent of the epidermis, hair, nails, and the organic matrix of the enamel of the teeth.

RECTAL ROUTE

Rectal administration of certain preparations can be used advantageously when the stomach is nonretentive or traumatized, when the medicine has an objectionable taste or odor, or when it can be changed by digestive enzymes. This route is also a reasonably convenient and safe method of giving drugs when the oral method is unsuitable, as when the patient is a small child or is unconscious.

Use of the rectal route avoids irritation of the upper gastrointestinal tract and may promote higher bloodstream drug titers because venous blood from the lower part of the rectum does not traverse the liver. The suppository drug vehicle is often superior to the retention enema vehicle because the drug is released at a slow but steady rate to ensure a protracted effect. Disadvantages of the retention enema are unpredictable retention of drug and the possibility of fluid passing above the lower rectum to be absorbed into the portal circulation, where metabolism can be extensive.

PARENTERAL ROUTE

The term **parenteral** means to be administered by injection. The four most common methods by which drugs are administered parenterally are **intradermal, subcutaneous, intramuscular,** and **intravenous** (Table 7-1). The medical imaging technologist may also witness intraarterial injections with certain medical procedures.

Parenteral administration of drugs includes all forms of drug injection into body tissues or fluids using a syringe and needle or catheter and container. Drugs given parenterally must be sterile, readily soluble and absorbable, and relatively nonirritating. Parenteral administration can be the most hazardous route by which to give a drug. Administering via this route requires specialized knowledge, aseptic technique, and manual skill to ensure safety and therapeutic effectiveness. Aseptic technique, accurate drug dosage, and proper technique and rate of injection at the proper site of injection are all essential to avoiding harm such as **lipodystrophy** (atrophy or hypertrophy of subcutaneous fat tissue), abscesses, necrosis, skin slough, nerve injuries, prolonged pain, or periostitis. *An injected drug acts rapidly and is irretrievable.* Thus, an error in dosage, method, or site is not easily corrected.

Routes of Drug Administration

Table 7-1 Suggested Injection Guidelines

Route	Common areas	Region	Needle sizes*	Volume injected (ml) Average	Range†	Examples of medications by this route
Intradermal (intracutaneous)	Skin (corium)	Inner aspect of midforearm or scapula	26 or 27 gauge × 3/8 in	0.1	0.001 to 1.0	Tuberculin, allergens, local anesthetics
Subcutaneous	Beneath the skin	Lateral upper arms; thighs; abdominal fat pads except the 1-in area around umbilicus and tissue over bone; upper back, upper hips	25 to 27 gauge × 1/2 to 5/8 in‡	0.5	0.5 to 1.5	Epinephrine (non-oily), insulin, some narcotics, tetanus toxoid, vaccines, vitamin B$_{12}$, heparin
Intramuscular	Gluteus medius	Dorsogluteal	20 to 23 gauge × 1½ to 3 in‡	2 to 4	1 to 5	Most intramuscular and Z-track injections
	Gluteus minimus	Ventrogluteal	20 to 23 gauge × 1½ to 3	1 to 4	1 to 5	All intramuscular medications
	Vastus lateralis	Anterolateral midthigh	22 to 25 gauge × 5/8 to 1 in‡	1 to 4	1 to 5	Almost all intramuscular medications
	Deltoid	Upper arm below shoulder	23 to 25 gauge × 5/8 to 1 in‡	0.5	0.5 to 2	Vaccines, absorbed tetanus toxoid, most narcotics, epinephrine, sedatives, vitamin B$_{12}$, lidocaine
Intravenous bolus	Cephalic and basilic veins	Dorsum of hand and forearm; antecubital fossa	18 to 23 gauge × 1 to 1½ in	1 to 10	0.5 to 50 (or more by continuous infusion)	Antibiotics, vitamins, fluids and electrolytes, antineoplastics, vasopressors, corticosteroids, aminophylline, blood products

*Needles used for withdrawing medication from a container should be changed before injecting medication drawn (1) from ampules, because irritating medication may cling to needle (filter-needles should be used to withdraw medication from ampules) and (2) from vials, because needles are dulled after insertion through rubber tops; disposable needles are thus labeled "for one-time use only."

†Administration of the largest volumes listed here should be avoided if possible by dividing the dose and using different sites or by using another route in consultation with prescriber.

‡See text for discussion of factors influencing choice of needle length.

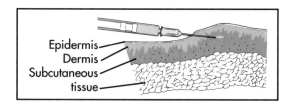

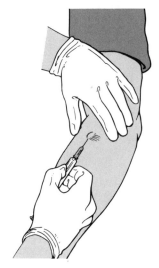

Fig. 7-1   Intradermal injection method. The needle penetrates epidermis and goes into dermis but not subcutaneous tissue. (Note that the skin is not pinched up.)

Most methods of parenteral administration may be performed by the technologist, but some are usually performed only by a physician or a nurse. Knowledge of, and strict adherence to, agency policy is imperative.

Intradermal (ID) Method

Intradermal or intracutaneous injection means that the injection is made into the upper layers of the skin almost parallel to the skin surface (Fig. 7-1).

The amount of drug given is small, and absorption is slow. This method is used mostly in testing for allergic reactions and for giving small amounts of a local anesthetic. In testing for allergic reactions, minute amounts of the solution to be tested are injected just under the outer layers of skin. The medial surface of the forearm and the skin of the back are sites frequently used. These injections are best made with a fine, short needle (26 or 27 gauge) and a small-barrel syringe (such as a tuberculin syringe) (Fig. 7-2).

Subcutaneous (SC) Method

Small amounts of drug in solution are given subcutaneously (beneath the layers of skin, yet above the muscle), usually by means of a 25-gauge (or thinner) needle and syringe. The needle is inserted through the skin with a quick movement, but the injection is made slowly and steadily (Fig. 7-3). The technologist should slightly withdraw the plunger of the

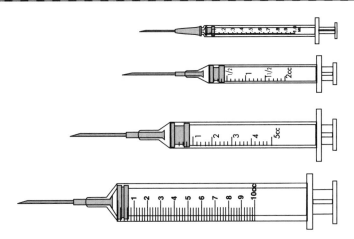

Fig. 7-2   Syringe types. These syringes are used to accurately measure varying amounts of liquids and liquid medications. The uppermost syringe is known as a tuberculin syringe and is graduated in 0.01 cc (ml). It is a syringe of choice for administration of very small amounts. The 2 cc syringe is the one commonly used to give a drug subcutaneously or intramuscularly. It is graduated in 0.1 cc. The larger syringes are used when a larger volume of drug is to be administered intramuscularly or intravenously; for withdrawing blood for laboratory testing; or for obtaining urine specimens from urinary catheters (20 cc syringes may be preferred for the last two uses). These syringes and needles are not drawn to scale (e.g., the tuberculin syringe is much thinner and shorter than the others).

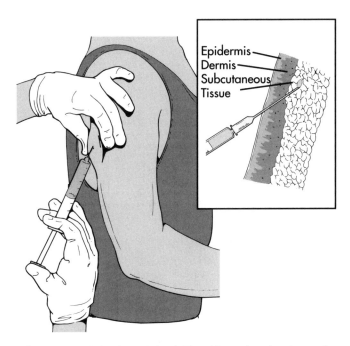

Fig. 7-3   Subcutaneous injection method. The skin surface has been cleansed, and the syringe is held at the angle at which the needle will penetrate subcutaneous tissue. The left hand is used to pinch the arm gently but firmly. When the needle has been inserted into the subcutaneous tissue, the tissue of the arm is released and the solution is steadily injected. Based on the patient's condition or the medication to be injected, judgment may dictate a different angle or an approach different from pinching up the skin.

syringe (aspirate) before injecting the drug, to make sure that a blood vessel has not been entered. If a red streak is observed as the plunger is withdrawn, the operator should assume that a vessel has been tapped. It is then necessary to reposition and/or replace the needle and possibly the syringe and contents. If this simple precaution is not observed, a subcutaneous injection immediately turns into an intravenous or intraarterial injection; either of which can be extremely dangerous to the patient (e.g., air embolism, hematoma, extravasation). The angle of insertion should usually be 45 to 60 degrees (but can vary between 30 and 90 degrees, depending on needle length and depth of fat pads. Insertion should be made on the fat pads of the abdomen, the outer surface of the upper arm, the anterior surface of the thigh, or occasionally the lower abdominal surface (when heparin is ordered). In these locations there are fewer large blood vessels, and sensation is less keen than on the medial surfaces of the extremities. Massage of the part after injection tends to increase the rate of absorption but should be avoided after injection of some drugs, such as heparin, to minimize bruising as the drug spreads through the tissues. Disposable syringes and needles contribute to aseptic safety of the procedure but also to cost and problems of storage and disposal. Subcutaneously injected medicines are limited to drugs that are highly soluble and nonirritating and to solutions of limited volume (ideally no more than 1 ml).

Irritating drugs given subcutaneously can result in the formation of sterile abscesses and necrotic tissue, especially if injections are made repeatedly in the same site. Care should be exercised to avoid contamination and to rotate sites. Subcutaneous injections are not effective in individuals with sluggish peripheral circulation (e.g., the patient in shock).

Intramuscular (IM) Method

Deeper injections are made into muscular tissue, through the skin and subcutaneous tissue, when a drug is too irritating to be given subcutaneously, although irritation may also occur with some drugs given intramuscularly. Larger doses can be given by intramuscular injection (up to 5 ml) than by subcutaneous injection. In cases of circulatory collapse (i.e., shock), intravenous injection is preferred over the *delayed* absorption via the SC, IM, or ID route.

A drug may be given intramuscularly in an **aqueous solution,** an **aqueous suspension,** or a solution or suspension of oil. Suspensions form a supply of drug in the tissue, and result in slow, gradual absorption. Two disadvantages sometimes encountered when preparations in oil are used are that the patient may be sensitive to the oil and the oil may not be absorbed. In the latter case, incision and drainage of the oil may be necessary. Fortunately, few drugs are formulated in oil.

Criteria for selection of a safe intramuscular injection site include distance from large, vulnerable nerves, bones, and blood vessels and from bruised, scarred, or swollen previous injection or infusion sites. The type of needle used for IM injection depends on the site of the in-

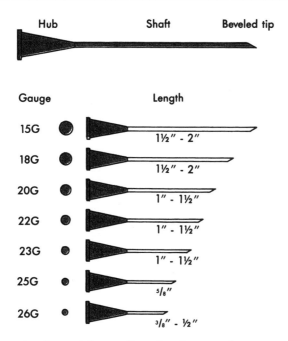

Fig. 7-4 Parts of the needle and various needle gauges.

jection, the condition of the tissues, the size of the patient, and the nature of the drug to be injected. Needles from 1 to 1½ inches in length are common. The usual **gauge** is 21 to 23 *(the larger the number, the finer the needle).* (See Fig. 7-4.) Fine needles can be used for thin solutions and heavier needles for suspensions and oils. Needles for injection into the deltoid area should be ⅝ to 1 inch in length, the gauge again depending on the material to be injected. The deltoid can readily absorb up to 2 ml of drug. For many IM injections the gluteals are preferred because of fewer nerve endings and less discomfort. The needle must be long enough to avoid depositing the solution of drug into the subcutaneous or fatty tissue. The depth of insertion depends on the amount of subcutaneous tissue and will vary with the weight of the patient.

It is essential to locate the appropriate landmarks to determine the areas safe for injections (Table 7-1 and Fig. 7-5). IM injections may be given into such clearly defined areas of musculature as the gluteal region of the lower back (provides slowest absorption), the deltoid area, and the anterolateral thigh. At first it seems to most students that the fleshy part of the buttock is a logical intramuscular site. It is not, since underneath, centrally, and running diagonally is the sciatic nerve, which if damaged can result in permanent leg paralysis. Every attempt must be made to avoid this area.

There are now two acceptable ways to map appropriate IM sites in the gluteal region. The formerly used method of dividing the gluteus medius into imaginary quadrants and injecting into the upper outer quadrant is out of favor because it does not necessarily prevent an injection into the sciatic nerve, especially if its course runs abnormally.

Table 7-2   Commonly Used Weights and Measures

Metric	Apothecary	Household
WEIGHT		
1 kg*	2.2 pounds	
1000 mg = 1 gram*	gr xv	
60 mg* (occasionally seen as 65 mg)	gr î	
30 mg	gr ss (one half)	
1 μg (mcg) = 0.001 mg		
VOLUME		
	4 quarts	1 gallon
1000 ml* = approx 1 liter = 1000 cc	Approx 1 qt	1 quart
500 ml	Approx 1 pint (½ qt)	16 ounces
240 or 250 ml	℥ viii (8 fluidounces)† = approx ½ pint	1 cup or 1 glass
30 ml* = approx 30 cc	℥ î (1 fluidounce)	2 tbsp
Approx 16 ml = approx 16 cc	ʒ iv (4 fluidrams)	1 tbsp
Approx 8 ml	ʒ îi (2 fluidrams)	2 tsp
4 to 5 ml	ʒ î (1 fluidram)	1 tsp
1 ml* = approx 1 cc	Minims xv or xvi	Minims cannot be compared with drops

*These equivalents may be committed to memory for ready application to dosage problems.
†Note the small difference in the symbols for fluidounce and fluidram.

The technologist can best locate the **dorsogluteal** site (the muscle underneath is the gluteus medius) by asking the patient to lie face down and exposing the entire area so that the landmarks and the injection site can be clearly located. The proper site for this injection is outlined by an imaginary diagonal line drawn from the area of the greater trochanter of the femur to the posterior iliac spine. The injection should be given at any point between that imaginary straight line and below the curve of the iliac crest (see Fig. 7-5, *A*).

The **ventrogluteal** site can be made accessible with the patient lying in a supine or side-lying position. This site is used for IM injections in either children or adults and could be used more often. To locate it on the left side, the technologist should palpate for the left greater trochanter with the right palm, point the right index finger to the anterior superior iliac spine, and extend the middle finger toward the iliac crest. The injection should be made into the center of the V formed between the index and middle fingers (see Fig. 7-5, *B*). The left hand is used to detect landmarks in the right hip.

The *mid-deltoid* area is the muscular area in the arm formed by the rectangle bounded on the top by the edge of the shoulder and on the

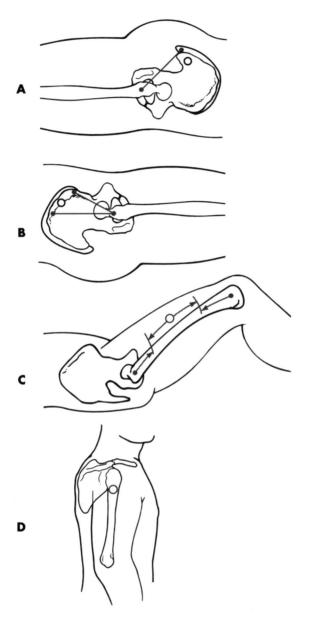

Fig. 7-5 Intramuscular injection sites. **A,** Dorsogluteal site, located anterior to the diagonal line from the trochanter to the posterior iliac spine. An injection near the middle of the buttocks may result in an injury to the sciatic nerve. The needle is inserted with a quick firm movement, entering perpendicular to the skin. After aspiration to make certain the needle is not in a blood vessel, the solution is injected slowly and steadily. **B,** Ventrogluteal intramuscular injection site. The V fans out from the greater trochanter between the anterior iliac spine and iliac crest. The injection site (O) is centered at the base of the triangle. **C,** Vastus lateralis (midlateral thigh) intramuscular injection site—a handsbreadth below the greater trochanter and a handsbreadth above the knee and halfway between the front and side of the thigh. **D,** Mid-deltoid intramuscular injection site—below the acromion and lateral to the axilla.

bottom by the beginning of the axilla (see Fig. 7-5, *D*). The deltoid muscle has a considerably higher blood flow than the other IM injection sites and, for rapid onset, is the area of choice for many small-volume (2 ml or less) medications.

The *vastus lateralis* is a muscular area in the upper outer leg. The potential area for injection is a long rectangular area just lateral to the frontal plane of the thigh. Its top boundary is found about one handsbreadth below the greater trochanter, and the bottom boundary is about one handsbreadth above the knee (see Fig. 7-5, *C*). This area can accommodate volumes of medication the same size as the gluteus medius and is distant from any major blood vessels or nerves. However, injection here may be more painful than in the buttocks.

For the IM injection, the needle and syringe assembly is held as if it were a dart while the other hand stretches the skin of the injection site taut. If the muscle mass underlying the injection site is inadequate to accommodate the length of the needle, the flesh may instead be pinched up before needle insertion. The injection should be made *perpendicular to the skin surface,* from a distance of about 2 inches, in one quick motion. If possible, the needle should not be inserted to its full depth and a small portion of needle should be left accessible above the skin so that the needle might be retrieved should it break, a very rare occurrence. As in subcutaneous injection, it is necessary to make certain that the needle is not in a blood vessel, thus causing the unintended deposit of medication into the bloodstream instead of muscle tissue. This is ascertained by pulling out the plunger *slightly* after the needle is in place in the tissue **(aspiration).** A slight pinkish tinge to the medication may be seen close to the needle hub or a small amount of blood may enter the barrel of the syringe, if the needle is in a blood vessel rather than in tissue. If this is the case, both needle and medication-filled syringe should be withdrawn and discarded before continuing. In certain cases, injection of oily or particulate medicines or bacteria by such an inadvertent intravascular administration could result in a serious emergency situation.

Contrary to popular belief, needle puncture of the skin is not always the prime source of discomfort associated with injections, although a dull needle such as one that has been inserted through a vial's rubber stopper will certainly contribute to pain. Also, it is not the length of the needle that causes pain, but the diameter; a 3-inch needle will hurt no more than a ⅝-inch one if the diameter is similar. Except for the psychologic aspect of anxiety about needles, most injection pain is thought to occur from stretching of tissue (pain receptors in the skin) as it accommodates the volume of the drug; from irritation from the drug itself; from unsteadiness in the injector's technique, which results in jiggling of the needle during overly slow insertions; during aspiration; while the injector is reaching for the antiseptic swab at completion; or from wet antiseptic on the skin during insertion. Firm pressure applied to the needle-tissue juncture with an antiseptic swab will prevent discomfort as the needle is withdrawn. Massaging the site acts to disperse the medication and may also reduce discomfort.

Intravenous (IV) Method

Because of the importance of intravenous injection techniques to the medical imaging technologist, Chapter 9 will be mostly dedicated to this subject.

GENERAL ADMINISTRATION GUIDELINES

The following are recommended guidelines for distributing or administering drugs to patients. Accurate and full identification of the patient prior to giving medications ensures that the right person gets the right medication. Remember the five rights of drug administration.

1. When preparing or giving medicines, focus all of your attention on the task. Do not permit yourself to be distracted while working with medicines.

2. Make certain that you have a written order for every medication for which you assume the responsibility of administration. (Verbal and telephone orders should be written out and signed by the prescriber as soon as possible. These orders should be used only in limited circumstances and not for the convenience of the prescriber.)

3. Make a habit of reading the label of the medicine and comparing it to the requisition carefully at least three times: first, when removing the drug from the supply drawer or medication cart; second, when placing the medication in a cup or syringe; and, third, just before administering it to the patient, before the container is discarded.

4. Never give a medicine from an unlabeled container or from one on which the label is not legible.

5. If you must in some way calculate the dosage for a client from the preparation on hand and you are uncertain of your calculation, verify your work on paper by having some other responsible person (i.e., instructor, lead technologist, pharmacist) check it. Whenever the result of a calculation calls for more than two units of a drug to make a dose, double-check the calculation. It is highly unusual for more than two units of a drug to be administered in a single dose.

6. When measuring liquids, hold the container so that the line indicating the desired quantity is on a level with the eye. The quantity is read when the lowest part of the concave surface of the fluid is on this line (i.e., the miniscus).

7. Dosage forms such as tablets, capsules, and pills should be handled so that the fingers do not come into contact with the medicine. Use the cap of the container to guide or lift the medicine into the medicine glass or container that you will be taking to the patient.

8. Avoid wasting medicines. Medicines tend to be expensive; in some instances a single capsule may cost the patient several dollars.

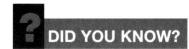

DID YOU KNOW?

Anytime a drug is administered to a patient, relevant information must be recorded on the patient's chart to document the event. The name and dosage of the drug, route of administration, date, time, and site of injection (if the drug is administered parenterally) should be included.

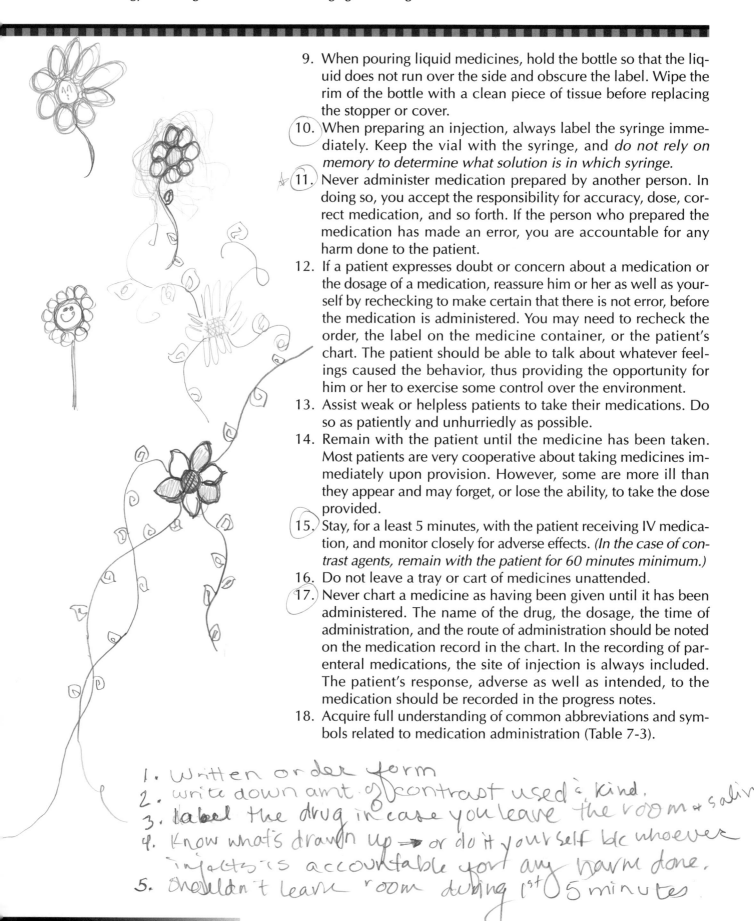

9. When pouring liquid medicines, hold the bottle so that the liquid does not run over the side and obscure the label. Wipe the rim of the bottle with a clean piece of tissue before replacing the stopper or cover.

10. When preparing an injection, always label the syringe immediately. Keep the vial with the syringe, and *do not rely on memory to determine what solution is in which syringe.*

11. Never administer medication prepared by another person. In doing so, you accept the responsibility for accuracy, dose, correct medication, and so forth. If the person who prepared the medication has made an error, you are accountable for any harm done to the patient.

12. If a patient expresses doubt or concern about a medication or the dosage of a medication, reassure him or her as well as yourself by rechecking to make certain that there is not error, before the medication is administered. You may need to recheck the order, the label on the medicine container, or the patient's chart. The patient should be able to talk about whatever feelings caused the behavior, thus providing the opportunity for him or her to exercise some control over the environment.

13. Assist weak or helpless patients to take their medications. Do so as patiently and unhurriedly as possible.

14. Remain with the patient until the medicine has been taken. Most patients are very cooperative about taking medicines immediately upon provision. However, some are more ill than they appear and may forget, or lose the ability, to take the dose provided.

15. Stay, for a least 5 minutes, with the patient receiving IV medication, and monitor closely for adverse effects. *(In the case of contrast agents, remain with the patient for 60 minutes minimum.)*

16. Do not leave a tray or cart of medicines unattended.

17. Never chart a medicine as having been given until it has been administered. The name of the drug, the dosage, the time of administration, and the route of administration should be noted on the medication record in the chart. In the recording of parenteral medications, the site of injection is always included. The patient's response, adverse as well as intended, to the medication should be recorded in the progress notes.

18. Acquire full understanding of common abbreviations and symbols related to medication administration (Table 7-3).

1. Written order form
2. Write down amt. of contrast used & kind.
3. Label the drug in case you leave the room & saline
4. Know what's drawn up → or do it yourself b/c whoever injects is accountable for any harm done.
5. Shouldn't leave room during 1st 5 minutes

Table 7-3   Common Abbreviations and Symbols Related to Medication Administration

Abbreviation	Unabbreviated form	Meaning
a	ante	before
ac	ante cibum	before meals
ad lib	ad libitum	freely
AM	ante meridiem	morning
bid	bis in die	twice each day
c̄	cum	with
cap	capsule	capsule
cc, cm³	cubic centimeter	cubic centimeter (ml)
clt	client	client
D/C or DC	discontinue	terminate
elix	elixir	elixir
g, gm	gram	1000 milligrams
gr	grain	60 milligrams
gtt	guttae	drops
h, hr	hora	hour
hs	hora somni	at bedtime
IM	intramuscular	into a muscle
IV	intravenous	into a vein
IVPB	IV piggyback	secondary IV line
kg	kilogram	2.2 lb
KVO	keep vein open	very slow infusion rate
Ⓛ	left	left
L	liter	liter
μg, mcg	microgram	one millionth of a gram
mg	milligram	one thousandth of a gram
mEq	milliequivalent	the number of grams of solute dissolved in one milliliter of a *normal* solution
min or m	minim	minim ($\frac{1}{15}$ or $\frac{1}{16}$ ml)
ml, mL	milliliter	one thousandth of a liter
ng	nanogram	one billionth of a gram
ō	no or none	no or none
OD	oculus dexter	right eye
OS	oculus sinister	left eye
os	os	mouth
OTC	over-the-counter	nonprescription drug
OU	oculus uterque	each eye
pc	post cibum	after meals
PM	post meridiem	after noon
PO	per os	by mouth, orally
prn	pro re nata	according to necessity
pt	patient	patient
q	quaque	every
qd	quaque die	every day
qh	quaque hora	every hour
q4h, q4°	every 4 hours	every 4 hours around the clock
qid	quater in die	four times each day
qod	quaque aliem die	every other day

Continued

Table 7-3   Common Abbreviations and Symbols Related to Medication Administration—cont'd

Abbreviation	Unabbreviated form	Meaning
qs	quantum satis	sufficient quantity
Ⓡ	right	right
℞	receipt	take
s̄	sine	without
SL	sub linguam	under the tongue
SOS	si opus sit	if necessary
ss	semis	a half
stat	statim	at once
SC, SQ	subcutaneous	into subcutaneous tissue
tbsp	tablespoon	tablespoon (15 ml)
tid	ter in die	three times a day
TO	telephone order	order received over the telephone
tsp	teaspoon	teaspoon (4 to 5 ml)
U	unit	a dosage measure for insulin, penicillin, heparin
VO	verbal order	order received verbally
î, îî	one, two	one, two (as in "gr î," "gr îî")
ʒ	dram	4 or 5 ml
℥	ounce or fluid ounce	ounce (30 milliliters)
×	times	as in two times a week
>	greater than	greater than
<	less than	less than
=	equal to	equal to
↑, ╱	increase or increasing	increase or increasing
↓, ╱	decrease or decreasing	decrease or decreasing

Learning Exercises

Abbreviations

Spell out each of the abbreviations below.

1. SC: _subcutaneous_

2. IM: _intramuscular_

3. IV: _intravenous_

True-False

Circle T for true and F for false.

1. T (F) Only when a drug is initially administered to a patient should relevant information be recorded in the patient's chart.

2. (T) F If you administer medication prepared by another person, and that person has made an error, you are accountable for any harm done to the patient resulting from that error.

3. T (F) It is acceptable practice to record medication administration in patients' charts before the actual event to clear the paperwork out of the way and concentrate on the task.

4. T (F) It is not the diameter of a needle but the length and depth of insertion that causes pain.

5. (T) F Injections should be made perpendicular to the skin surface from a distance of about 2 inches, in one quick motion.

6. (T) F The mid-deltoid area is the muscular area in the arm formed by the rectangle bounded on the top by the edge of the shoulder and on the bottom by the beginning of the axilla.

7. (T) F Intramuscular injections are given when a drug is too irritating to be given subcutaneously.

8. T (F) Intradermal injections are given beneath the layers of skin and above the muscle.

Multiple-Choice Questions

Place a check before the letter of the correct answer.

1. What is the term for the administration of drugs placed under the tongue?

____ **a.** Sublingual
____ **b.** Topical
____ **c.** Parenteral
____ **d.** Subcutaneous

2. Which of the following statements expresses the correct relation between lumen diameter and gauge number?

____ **a.** As the diameter increases, the gauge number stays the same.
____ **b.** As the diameter increases, the gauge number increases.
____ **c.** As the diameter decreases, the gauge number increases.
____ **d.** As the diameter decreases, the gauge number decreases.

3. During intramuscular injections, it is necessary to determine if the needle is in a blood vessel. What is the term for the slight pulling of the syringe plunger to check for this dangerous problem?

____ **a.** Injection
____ **b.** Aspiration
____ **c.** Extravasation
____ **d.** Infiltration

4. Which of the following would not be considered one of the "five rights" of drug administration?

____ **a.** Right time
____ **b.** Right place
____ **c.** Right patient
____ **d.** Right drug

5. The abbreviation qh means that the drug should be delivered at what intervals?

____ **a.** Daily
____ **b.** Every 4 hours
____ **c.** Hourly
____ **d.** Every 2 hours

6. What is the term for injections made into the upper layers of skin, almost parallel to the skin surface?

____ **a.** Intramuscular
____ **b.** Intravenous
____ **c.** Topical
____ **d.** Intradermal

7. Tuberculin, allergens, and local anesthetics are best delivered via which route of injection?
   _____ **a.** Subcutaneous
   _____ **b.** Intradermal
   _____ **c.** Intramuscular
   _____ **d.** Intravenous

8. What is the term for a medication applied to the skin in order to decrease the number of microorganisms?
   _____ **a.** Astringent
   _____ **b.** Emollient
   _____ **c.** Antiseptic
   _____ **d.** Cleansing agent

9. When a drug is injected subcutaneously, what should be the angle of needle insertion?
   _____ **a.** 20 degrees
   _____ **b.** 45 to 60 degrees
   _____ **c.** 90 degrees
   _____ **d.** 120 degrees

10. What does the term parenteral mean?
   _____ **a.** Administration of a drug by mouth
   _____ **b.** Administration of a drug by injection
   _____ **c.** Assessment of patient history
   _____ **d.** Acquisition of consent for minors

Review Questions

1. What are the guidelines for administering drugs intramuscularly to patients? ① injection site far from nerves, bones, blood vessels, ② proper needle length + gauge ③ hold needle + pipe as if it were a dart ⊥ to site in 2" from skin ④ determine proper location ⑤ inject ⑥ massage site to disperse the drug

2. What are two acceptable ways for a technologist to map appropriate IM sites in the gluteal region? (Describe in detail.)
   ① Pt. lies face down or on side

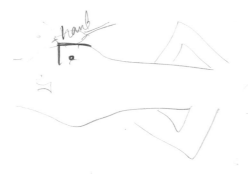

8

Infection Control

KEY TERMS

bacteria
body substance precautions (BSP)
conidia
cycle of infection
dimorphic
fomite
disinfection
fungi
human immunodeficiency virus (HIV)
medical asepsis
microbial dilution
microorganisms
nosocomial
pathogen
protozoa
reservoir of infection
sterilization
surgical asepsis
universal precautions
viruses

OBJECTIVES

At the conclusion of this chapter you should be able to:
1. Define medical asepsis, disinfection, and sterilization.
2. List four factors involved when pathogenic organisms are transferred from person to person.
3. State five examples of personal hygiene that help in preventing the spread of infection.
4. Demonstrate techniques for effective hand washing.
5. Describe the correct method of linen disposal using medical asepsis principles.
6. Demonstrate steps used in discarding disposable equipment in the clinical area.
7. Name the agent used for disinfecting equipment in the radiology department.

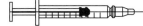

INTRODUCTION

Hospitals are assembly places for the sick and are, therefore, focal points for the transmission of infection. Anyone with a health problem is more susceptible to infection, and for this reason medical asepsis is of critical importance in patient care, especially when the imaging technologist is performing intravenous injection techniques.

Medical asepsis deals with reducing the *probability* of infectious organisms being transmitted to a susceptible individual. Any organism in an optimum environment will multiply at a rapid rate. Although the body has the ability to overcome a limited number of infectious organisms, this resistance can be overwhelmed by a massive exposure. Therefore, the fewer organisms to which a patient or health care worker is exposed, the better the chance of resisting infection. The process of reducing the number of organisms is called **microbial dilution** and can be accomplished at several levels.

Simple cleanliness measures avoid transmitting organisms by using proper cleaning, dusting, linen handling, and hand washing techniques. The second level is **disinfection** and involves the destruction of pathogens by using chemical materials. The third stage is **surgical asepsis** or **sterilization.** This involves treating items with heat, gas, or chemicals to make them germ free. They are then wrapped and stored in a manner that prevents contamination.

THE CYCLE OF INFECTION

The four factors involved in the spread of disease are sometimes called the **cycle of infection** (Fig. 8-1). For infections to be transmitted, there must first be an infectious organism, a reservoir of infection, a susceptible host, and a means of transporting the organism from the reservoir to the susceptible individual.

Infectious Organisms

Infectious organisms are too small to be seen with human vision and are referred to as **microorganisms.** They include bacteria, viruses, protozoa, and fungi.

> **Bacteria:** single-celled, procaryotic microorganisms that differ from all other organisms (the eukaryotes) in lacking a true nucleus and organelles such as mitochondria, chloroplasts, and lysosomes. Their genetic material consists of a single loop of double-stranded DNA, whereas the genetic material of eukaryotes consists of multiple chromosomes, which are complex structures of DNA and protein. Bacteria reproduce by cell division about every 20 minutes, giving them a very high rate of population growth and evolution. Some bacteria have the ability to produce a highly resistant resting form known as an *endospore.* These

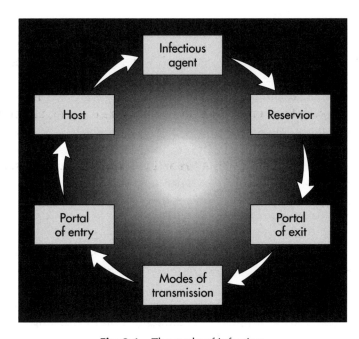

Fig. 8-1   The cycle of infection.

spores are extremely resistant to chemical and physical agents and are thus highly resistant to the external environment. They can remain viable for years and then germinate in response to specific environmental requirements.

Viruses: simpler in form compared with bacteria or animal cells. Viruses are neither procaryotic nor eukaryotic. They are considered obligate (unnecessary), intracellular parasites, which cannot live outside a living cell. They lack the components necessary for their own survival because of their inability to synthesize specific required proteins. Viruses carry their own genetic information in the form of DNA or RNA, but never both. The virus attaches to a host cell and inserts its genome or genetic information into the host. It then uses the organelles and metabolic functions of the host cell to produce new viruses. Once this process is completed, the new viral particles are released from the host, sometimes resulting in the destruction of the cell.

Protozoa: unicellular organisms that are neither plants nor animals and that can be ingested and transmitted through contaminated feces. They are distinguished from bacteria by their greater size and the fact that they do not possess a cell wall. They are motile, eukaryotic, sometimes parasitic organisms that are able to ingest food particles, and some even have simple digestive systems. Protozoa are classified according to their motility (amoeba-like, flagellate, ciliar, or nonmotile). Some protozoa are able to form *cysts,* which are resistant to chemical and physical changes, permitting them to survive while out of the host organism.

Fungi: can be macroscopic, as in the case of mushrooms and puffballs, or microscopic, such as yeasts and molds. They are eukaryotic organisms with a nucleus and membrane-bound organelles. Fungi are also much larger than bacteria. Medically important pathogenic fungi are **dimorphic.** That is, they have the ability to grow in two distinct forms, either as a single-celled yeast or as filamentous hyphae. Filamentous hyphae are better known as mold. Whether the organism is present in either form depends on the growth conditions. A photomicrograph of a typical mold would reveal a structure similar to that of a plant or a small tree. The molds produce tiny branches that extend into the air. It is here that spores are formed. These spores are called **conidia.** They are lightweight, resistant to drying, and easily dispersed to new environments.

Organisms capable of causing disease are called pathogenic organisms or **pathogens.** Some microorganisms live on or within the body as part of our normal flora. They aid in digestion and skin preservation and are nonpathogenic as long as they are confined to their usual environment. For example, *Candida albicans* may be found in the throat or gastrointestinal tract of many healthy individuals. Yet this organism often assumes a pathogenic role, causing urinary and vaginal infections in females and respiratory diseases in both males and females. See Table 8-1 for some common human pathogens.

Table 8-1 Some Examples of Pathogens

System	Name	Classification	Disease	Mode of transmission
Respiratory tract	*Bordetella pertussis*	Bacterium	Whooping cough	Airborne
	Candida albicans	Fungus	Pneumonia, thrush	Airborne
	Corynebacterium diphtheriae	Bacterium	Diphtheria	Airborne
	Influenza virus	Virus	Flu	Airborne and droplets
	Mycobacterium tuberculosis	Bacterium	Tuberculosis	Airborne and droplets
	Mumps virus	Virus	Mumps	Airborne
	Streptococcus pneumoniae	Bacterium	Pneumonia and sinus infections	Airborne
	Streptococcus pyogenes	Bacterium	Strep throat	Airborne
Gastrointestinal tract	*Entamoeba histolytica*	Protozoan	Amebic dysentery	Food, water
	Giardia lamblia	Protozoan	Giardiasis	Food, water
	Polio virus	Virus	Poliomyelitis	Food, water
	Salmonella species	Bacterium	Salmonellosis (food infection)	Food, water
	Shigella species	Bacterium	Shigellosis (bacillary dysentery)	Food, water
Genitourinary tract	*Escherichia coli*	Bacterium	Cystitis, nephritis	Contact
	Herpes simplex, 2	Virus	Genital herpes	Sexual contact
	Neisseria gonorrhoeae	Bacterium	Gonorrhea	Sexual contact
	Proteus species	Bacterium	Cystitis, nephritis	Contact
	Treponema pallidum	Bacterium	Syphilis	Sexual contact
	Trichomonas vaginalis	Protozoan	Vaginitis	Sexual contact
Skin	Herpes simplex, 1	Virus	Fever blisters	Contact, predisposition
	Measles virus	Virus	Measles	Airborne, contact
	Staphylococcus aureus	Bacterium	Boils, wound infections	Contact
	Tinea capitis	Fungus	Ringworm	Contact, predisposition
	Tinea pedis	Fungus	Athlete's foot	Contact, predisposition
Blood	*Borrelia burgdorferi*	Bacterium	Lyme disease	Vectors (ticks)
	Hepatitis B	Virus	Serum hepatitis	Contaminated serum
	Human immunodeficiency virus	Virus	AIDS	Mixing of human fluids
	Leptospira	Bacterium	Leptospirosis	Food, water, contact
	Plasmodium species	Sporozoan	Malaria	Vectors (mosquitoes)
	Salmonella typhi	Bacterium	Typhoid fever	Food, water

The Reservoir of Infection

The **reservoir,** or source, **of infection** may be any suitable place where pathogens can thrive in sufficient numbers to pose a threat. Such an environment must provide moisture, nutrients, and a suitable temperature, all of which are found in the human body. Thus, the source of infection might be a patient with hepatitis, a radiographer with an upper respiratory infection, or a linen handler with staphylococcic boils.

Since some pathogens live in the bodies of healthy individuals without causing apparent disease, it is quite possible for a person to be the reservoir for an infectious organism without realizing it. These persons are called "carriers." Many of us have throat cultures that are positive for *Staphylococcus aureus* without suffering from a sore throat. A susceptible patient with an open wound could contract a life-threatening infection if contaminated with this organism. The classic example of a carrier of infection is Typhoid Mary, a "healthy" food handler. Hundreds of cases of typhoid fever were attributed to contamination of the meals she helped to prepare. Today an example of a carrier of infection is the asymptomatic individual infected with **human immunodeficiency virus (HIV)** who spreads the disease through sexual intercourse or by sharing contaminated needles with intravenous drug users.

Although the human body is the most common reservoir of infection, any environment that will support the growth of microorganisms has the potential to be a secondary source. Such sources might include contaminated food or water or any damp, warm place that is not cleaned regularly.

The Susceptible Host

Susceptible hosts are quite frequently patients whose impaired health has reduced their natural resistance to infection. In addition to the primary problem that caused their hospitalization, they may develop a secondary infection. Mr. Grey, the postsurgical patient who develops an upper respiratory infection, or Mrs. Szekely, the medical patient with a urinary tract infection, may have **nosocomial,** or hospital-acquired, diseases.

Hospital-acquired infections also pose a threat to health care workers. In the United States, 8000 to 12,000 health care workers are infected with the hepatitis B virus (HBV) each year, resulting in 200 deaths. This particular strain of hepatitis is highly infectious, requires intensive treatment, and may lead to lifelong health problems. In 1991, the Occupational Safety and Health Administration (OSHA) published regulations requiring health care employers to provide HBV immunizations to employees, as well as procedures and equipment to prevent the transmission of HIV and other blood-borne diseases to which employees are exposed.

Hospital workers are exposed to a multitude of pathogens. In a single day, a medical imaging technologist may care for ambulatory outpatients, hospital isolation patients, and emergency trauma cases with "dirty" wounds. The technologist who works when his or her resistance is low as a result of fatigue, stress, or a low-grade infection has increased susceptibility as a host.

Transmission of Disease

The most direct way to intervene in the cycle of infection is to prevent transmission of the infectious organism from the reservoir to the susceptible host. To accomplish this successfully, it is first necessary to understand the four main routes of transmission.

The first route is by means of *direct contact.* This implies that the host is touched by an infected person and thus exposed to the pathogen.

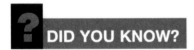

DID YOU KNOW?

Pathogens can leave the human body through a variety of means. The skin, mucous membranes, respiratory tract, gastrointestinal tract, surgical tubes and drains, urine, blood, and breaks in the skin allow pathogens to exit the body and infect susceptible hosts.

Syphilis is contracted when infectious organisms from the mucous membrane of one individual are placed in direct contact with the mucous membrane of a susceptible host. Skin infections are quite common among hospital workers because of the frequent contact with patients who have staphylococcic or herpetic diseases.

The three other principal routes of transmission are *indirect* and involve transport of organisms by means of fomites, vectors, and airborne contamination.

An object that has been in contact with pathogenic organisms is called a **fomite.** The contaminated urinary catheter that caused Mrs. Szekely's urinary tract infection is a good example. Other fomites in the radiology department might include the x-ray table, the CT or MRI patient couch, the chin-rest on the chest board, calipers, positioning sponges, the ultrasound transducer, the gamma camera surface, a mishandled syringe, and, especially, the technologist's hands.

A vector is an animal in which an infectious organism develops or multiplies before becoming infective to a new host. Some examples of vectors are mosquitoes that transmit malaria, fleas that harbor bubonic plaque, ticks that convey Lyme disease, and animals such as dogs, bats, or squirrels in which rabies is endemic. The bite of infected insects or mammals may thus transmit diseases to humans.

Airborne contamination is spread by means of droplets and dust. Droplet contamination often occurs when an infectious individual coughs, sneezes, or speaks in the vicinity of a susceptible host. Mr. Grey, for example, may have acquired his upper respiratory infection from the nurse who sneezed while preparing him for surgery.

Although many organisms are fragile, requiring continuous warmth, moisture, and nutrients to exist, others are capable of forming spores. In this stage, the organism is resistant to heat, cold, and drying and can live without nourishment. Spores can float through the air and lurk in dusty corners waiting to invade a susceptible host. Spore-forming organisms are responsible for such diseases as tetanus, anthrax, histotoxic infections (poisonous to tissues), gas gangrene, and septicemia. Recent epidemiologic studies have shown that some viruses, such as those causing oral and genital herpes, can resist drying for weeks. This should emphasize the need for practical asepsis.

PREVENTING DISEASE TRANSMISSION

At one time, cleanliness was the only defense against infection. We now live in an age that benefits from antibiotics that significantly reduce the suffering and death once caused by infections. However, do not be deluded into thinking that an antibiotic exists for every infectious disease. Viral infections are resistant to most antibiotics. Other organisms, such as staphylococci, apparently mutate rapidly, acquiring immunity against medications that were once highly effective. In any case, disease prevention is clearly preferable to the most efficient cure. Therefore, the practice of medical asepsis is still the first line of defense in preventing the spread of disease.

Historical Perspective

When infectious disease was rampant, infected persons were often "quarantined," which meant that members of a household were prevented from leaving their home and others were excluded to confine the infection to one family rather than spreading it through an entire community. Later, hospitals developed policies that involved separating patients admitted with infectious diseases from other patients. Contacts with other persons were rigidly controlled. This "isolation" was a logical outgrowth of the former practice of quarantine. These techniques provided for specialized methods of asepsis when the danger of disease transmission was exceptionally great.

Although isolation techniques were effective when used correctly, no mechanism existed for the prevention of serious diseases carried by asymptomatic individuals. This has certainly been true of patients who are carriers of HBV and those with HIV, the infectious agent responsible for AIDS.

HIV and AIDS

The rapid spread of HIV infection and AIDS is a source of concern to everyone. Of the estimated 1 million plus individuals in the United States infected with HIV, approximately 20% have developed AIDS. Since the undiagnosed HIV carrier may be asymptomatic for as long as 10 years, the potential for spreading disease assumes immense proportions. Of the first 100,000 cases reported, 61% occurred among homosexual or bisexual males with no history of being intravenous drug users (IDUs) and 20% among heterosexual male or female IDUs. More recent statistics show a dramatic increase in heterosexual transmission. It is expected that the rate for non-IDU heterosexual transmission will increase by more than 50% by the year 2000. Although drugs have been developed that prolong the time required for HIV infections to progress to AIDS, at this time no known cure exists. New vaccines have been developed but have not yet been tested and approved for use in the United States.

Fortunately, the AIDS virus is not acquired by casual contact (e.g., touching or shaking hands; eating food prepared by an infected person; contact with drinking fountains, telephones, toilets, or other surfaces). It is not an airborne disease. The routes of transmission are through sexual contact, from contaminated blood or needles, and to the fetus if the mother is infected.

Since AIDS is an immunodeficiency condition, the primary cause of death is a secondary disease or combination of diseases. Among the conditions frequently involved are Kaposi's sarcoma, *Pneumocystis carinii* pneumonia, and other opportunistic infections. One effect of the AIDS epidemic has been a sharp rise in the number of tuberculosis infections. As the incidence of drug-resistant tuberculosis continues to rise, an increasing number of these patients probably will be hospitalized for treatment.

As a health care worker, you must expect to encounter unidentified or undiagnosed patients with AIDS or HBV. Currently, controversy surrounds the patient's right to confidentiality regarding the AIDS diagnosis, even within the hospital setting. This may prevent you from being informed about diagnosed patients. Also, diagnosed patients are only the "tip of the iceberg." It is estimated that as many as 50 undiagnosed patients with serious viral disease exist for every known case. Anxiety about HIV infections is typical and understandable among health care workers. However, the occupational risk is not great. More than 95% of the health care workers infected with HIV were exposed as a result of activities unrelated to their work. The most common occupational exposure by far is the needle stick. Many thousands of needle sticks have been reported in the last 10 years, but fewer than 100 health care workers with no other identified risk factors have been diagnosed as HIV positive.

Universal Precautions

Since persons infected with AIDS, HBV, or other diseases (e.g., typhoid fever) may have no symptoms, you must treat all patients as potential reservoirs of infection.

The Centers for Disease Control (CDC) is now recommending a system of infection control called **body substance precautions (BSP),** or **universal precautions.** This system is based on the use of barriers for all contacts with all body substances rather than focusing on the isolation of a patient with a diagnosed disease. The need to use barriers such as gloves and masks depends on the nature of the interaction with the patient rather than on the specific diagnosis. Emphasis is placed on all body fluids being potential sources of infection, regardless of diagnosis.

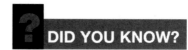
DID YOU KNOW?

Each time you come in contact with patients, if you do not wash your hands, or remove or change gloves, the patient's infectious organisms have just relocated to the control panel or console you are about to come in contact with. Think about it.

UNIVERSAL PRECAUTIONS

1. Gloves should be worn when you are in contact with blood, body fluids containing visible blood, mucous membranes, or nonintact skin.
2. Gloves should be worn when you are handling items or touching surfaces soiled with blood or body fluids or when performing venipuncture or other vascular access procedures.
3. Gloves should be changed after contact with each patient.
4. Masks and protective eye shields should be worn during procedures that can generate droplets of blood or other body fluids, to prevent exposure of mucous membranes of the mouth, nose, and eyes to infection.
5. Gowns should be worn during procedures that can result in the splashing of blood or other body fluids.
6. Hands and other skin surfaces should be thoroughly washed immediately after contamination with blood or body fluids.
7. Needles should not be recapped, purposely bent or broken, or removed from syringes.
8. Needles and syringes must be disposed of in puncture-resistant containers in the immediate work area.
9. Mouthpieces, Ambu-bags, and ventilation devices should be used rather than mouth-to-mouth resuscitation.
10. Health care workers with oozing or open sores should refrain from direct contact and handling of patient care equipment or items.

Although this system was not developed solely in response to the AIDS epidemic, it does meet all criteria for dealing with these patients, as well as those with other viral diseases and certain bacterial diseases for which no effective antibiotic may exist. Using a BSP program discourages transmission from patient to patient as well as from patient to caregiver. The key to effective protection is a consistent approach to *all* contact with *all* body substances of *all* patients at *all* times.

MEDICAL ASEPSIS

It is easy to find examples of poor aseptic technique in most clinical settings. Unfortunately, the results of carelessness are seldom traced to the person responsible. It is the patient acquiring a nosocomial infection who suffers. Armed with the knowledge of disease transmission routes, health care workers can fight the spread of disease through the following steps:
1. Stay home when ill.
2. Cover mouth and nose when coughing or sneezing.
3. Wear a clean uniform or surgical scrubs daily, and remove it (if possible) prior to going home.
4. Wash hands often and use good housekeeping techniques.
5. Use BSP when handling linens or items contaminated with body substance.

Hand Washing

The first three principles are so simple as to be self-explanatory. Hand washing may also seem obvious, but this is the one rule most consistently ignored in most patient settings. Medically aseptic hand washing technique is both simple and effective. It should be followed explicitly before and after work and any time the hands have been heavily contaminated. Since a technologist's duties frequently demand brief contacts with a series of patients, it is especially important to *wash hands between patients* (Fig. 8-2). The Centers for Disease Control has established the following hand washing guidelines for health care workers. Wash hands in the following situations:
1. Before contact with patients (especially if they are highly susceptible to infection)
2. After caring for infected patients
3. After touching any organic material
4. Before performing invasive procedures such as IV injections, suctioning, and bladder catheterization
5. Before and after handling dressings or touching open wounds
6. After handling contaminated equipment
7. Before preparing medications
8. Between contacts with different patients, especially those in high-risk units such as critical care and nursery units
9. After using the restroom
10. After sneezing, coughing, or blowing your nose
11. After removing your gloves

1. Turn the water to the desired flow and temperature.
2. Wet your hands and lower your arms completely under the running water, holding hands and forearms lower than your elbows.
3. Apply a generous amount of soap to hands (1 to 2 ml).
4. Lather well (10 to 15 seconds), using friction to loosen and remove dirt and bacteria. Interlace fingers and rub palms and back of hands in a circular motion at least 5 times.
5. Use an orangewood stick to clean under and around your fingernails, being careful not to tear or cut your

skin. If you wear artificial nails, spend extra time washing your hands because artificial nails may harbor more bacteria.
6. Rinse your hands and wrists thoroughly, allowing water to run from wrists to fingertips.
7. Using a paper towel, dry your hands thoroughly from fingertips to wrists and forearms. Discard the paper towel in the proper receptacle.
8. Turn the water off using foot or knee controls or a clean paper towel on hand faucet controls.

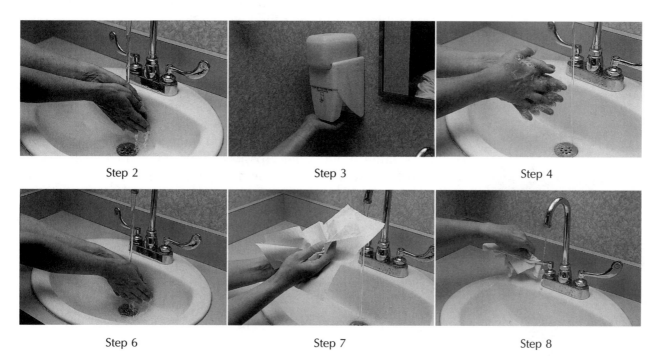

Step 2   Step 3   Step 4

Step 6   Step 7   Step 8

Fig. 8-2   Hand washing technique.

Housekeeping

Good housekeeping also reduces the incidence of airborne infections and the transfer of pathogens by fomites. A clean, dry environment discourages the growth of all microorganisms. Much of the cleaning in the radiology department may be done at night by the housekeeping staff, but the technologist is responsible for inspecting the work area regularly and maintaining high standards of medical asepsis.

Several general principles apply whenever cleaning is required. Always clean from the least contaminated area toward the more contaminated area and from the top down. Avoid raising dust, and do not contaminate yourself or clean areas.

One of the technologist's primary duties is to clean the patient table, couch, or cart between examinations. Use a cloth moistened with disinfectant such as Cidex, Staphene, Lysol, or Clorox. The CDC recommends sodium hypochlorite bleach (Clorox) as the preferred disin-

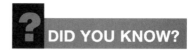

DID YOU KNOW?

In a recent study, physicians were listed *number one* as the health professionals least likely to wash their hands between patient contacts. *Number two* on the list were *radiologic technologists.*

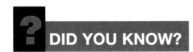

DID YOU KNOW?

Biopsies and other surgical procedures are no longer performed only in a surgical or angiography suite. It is becoming more and more common for MRI, CT, mammography, sonography, and even nuclear medicine technologists to be involved with surgical procedures. A working knowledge of surgical aspepsis has never been more important in these areas.

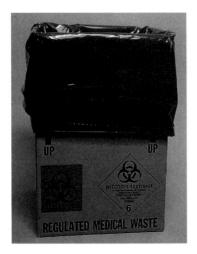

Fig. 8-3 Biohazardous waste container and symbol.

fectant for preventing the spread of HIV. If using Clorox, mix it daily in a 1:10 solution because the effectiveness declines rapidly.

Every piece of equipment that comes in contact with the patient, such as the chest film holder or the gamma camera, must also be cleaned after each use. Most hospitals have written procedures with detailed instructions concerning preferred cleansing agents and the extent of responsibility for disinfecting rooms.

Handling Linens

Linens may become dangerous fomites if proper aseptic technique is not observed. Objects or linens soiled with body secretions (mucus, vomitus, urine, feces) are considered contaminated, even though stains may not be apparent. Any linens used by patients should be handled as little as possible. To prevent airborne contamination, fold the edges of linens to the middle without shaking or flapping. Immediately place loosely balled linens in a hamper. *Never* use any linen for more than one patient.

The uniform should be protected with a gown while assisting incontinent patients or helping to clean up trauma patients. For the protection of laundry workers, grossly contaminated linens should be placed in a separate plastic bag and marked, for example, "Fecal Contamination." Many hospitals provide laundry bags that dissolve in hot water. This reduces the number of times linen must be handled and helps protect the laundry personnel in particular.

The floor is always considered grossly contaminated, and anything touching it is disposed of immediately. This includes linens as well as instruments and other items. When in doubt as to the cleanliness of any object, do not use it.

Disposal of Contaminated Waste

A modern hospital uses many disposable items, from simple objects such as paper cups and tissues to more complex items such as catheterization sets. *Disposable items are designed to be used only once and then discarded.* The only exception to this rule involves the immediate reuse of an unsterile item (e.g., emesis basin) by the same patient.

Each hospital has a routine for the discarding of disposable items. Some separate glass, plastic, and paper into covered containers. Others place everything together. Recent regulations demand that objects contaminated with blood or body fluids be discarded in a suitable container and marked with the biohazard symbol (see Fig. 8-3).

Needles and syringes are disposed of in special containers designed to receive the syringe without recapping it with the needle cover (Fig. 8-4). If a needle *must* be recapped (e.g., the container is too far away, or the patient cannot be left alone), place the cover on a hard surface and insert the needle without using the other hand. If needles are frequently recapped, it is helpful to have a needle cap holder attached to the counter in the work area. This holds the cap upright for one-handed needle insertion. *Most finger punctures occur during recapping of a needle.*

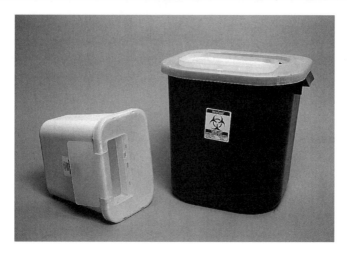

Fig. 8-4 Puncture-proof containers for needle and syringe disposal.

Be careful not to prick your finger. An accidental needle prick or skin broken by a contaminated object may be cause for concern. If this occurs, an incident report must be filed even though the injury seems insignificant. In addition to an incident report, most hospitals now ask that a baseline blood sample be drawn. Since HIV infection will not be apparent in the blood for approximately 3 months, this helps rule out infection acquired before the occupational exposure. After 3 to 4 months, another blood sample is tested for HIV.

Bandages and dressing should be handled with gloves and should be placed directly into waterproof bags, which should be sealed before discarding.

Always wear gloves when assisting patients with bedpans or urinals. Be sure to empty them at once, unless a specimen is needed. Rinse them well over the hopper or toilet, and discard or put them in the proper place to be sterilized unless they are to be reused immediately by the same patient.

Learning Exercises

Abbreviations

Spell out each of the abbreviations below.

1. CDC:

2. BSP:

3. IDU:

4. HBV:

5. OSHA:

True-False

Circle T for true and F for false.

1. **T** **F** Infectious organisms too small to be seen with unaided human vision are called microorganisms and include bacteria, viruses, protozoans, and fungi.

2. **T** **F** Some pathogens aid in digestion and skin preservation.

3. **T** **F** The human body is the most common reservoir of infection; however, secondary sources include contaminated food or water or any damp, warm place that is not regularly cleaned.

4. **T** **F** Since technologists are exposed to many pathogens during the course of a day, the technologist who works when his or her resistance is low because of fatigue, stress, or a low-grade infection has increased susceptibility as a host.

5. **T** **F** Three routes of transmission of infection are direct and involve transport of organisms by means of fomites, vectors, and airborne contamination.

6. T F   When treating patients with serious diseases, the symptoms will be readily apparent to you. You should take extra safety precautions with these patients.

7. T F   Proper hand washing is important after handling dressings or touching open wounds, but not necessarily before.

8. T F   Radiologic technologists, along with physicians, are often offenders when it comes to not washing their hands between patients.

Multiple-Choice Questions

Place a check before the letter of the correct answer.

1. Microorganisms causing infectious diseases are classified as which of the following?
_____ **a.** Lytic
_____ **b.** Endogenous
_____ **c.** Pathogenic
_____ **d.** Nosocomial

2. Which of the following is not a type of indirect disease transmission?
_____ **a.** Vector
_____ **b.** Fomite
_____ **c.** Aerosol
_____ **d.** Touching

3. The common cold is an example of an infection by which of the following?
_____ **a.** Bacteria
_____ **b.** Virus
_____ **c.** Fungus
_____ **d.** Protozoa

4. What term best describes the absolute removal of all life forms?
_____ **a.** Disinfection
_____ **b.** Medical asepsis
_____ **c.** Antisepsis
_____ **d.** Sterilization

5. A health care worker is accidentally punctured with a contaminated needle. This type of transmission is known as which of the following?
_____ **a.** Iatrogenic
_____ **b.** Vector
_____ **c.** Fomite
_____ **d.** Nosocomial

6. What is the most common means of spreading infection?
   ____ a. Improperly disposed of contaminated waste
   ____ b. Instruments improperly sterilized
   ____ c. Soiled linen
   ____ d. Human hands

7. What is the preferred disinfectant used to prevent the spread of HIV?
   ____ a. Iodine
   ____ b. Clorox
   ____ c. Lysol
   ____ d. Cidex

8. Tetanus is actually caused by which of the following?
   ____ a. Bacteria
   ____ b. Virus
   ____ c. Spore-forming organism
   ____ d. Nosocomial infection

9. What is the term for objects that have been in contact with pathogenic organisms?
   ____ a. Fomites
   ____ b. Pathogens
   ____ c. Microbes
   ____ d. Viruses

Review Questions

1. Why is it never good practice to recap needles?

2. What are five of the 10 Universal Precautions issued by the CDC?

Intravenous Drug Administration Technique (Venipuncture)

9

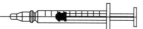

INTRODUCTION

Once the imaging technologist has a firm grasp of medical asepsis, the techniques involving **venipuncture** may be described, practiced, and mastered.

Intravenous (IV) fluids and medications are administered to meet specific needs. This route of drug administration allows patients to respond rapidly to medication. The IV injection is used for delivering most emergency medications when an immediate response is critical.

Dehydrated patients may need fluid and electrolyte replacement. The most common replacement fluids are normal saline and a 5% solution of dextrose in water. These solutions are usually stocked in radiology departments. If you are starting or replacing IV fluids, be certain that the solution is correct. Less common solutions or those containing medication may need to be replaced by the nursing or pharmacy service.

The IV route may serve to transport parenteral nutrition or chemotherapy. This is also the route used to inject ROCM in radiographic examinations of the urinary tract and in some CT studies, for MRI contrast agents, to inject radioactive nuclides in nuclear medicine, and to provide sedation during invasive procedures and MRI examinations.

IV EQUIPMENT

Venipuncture may be accomplished with a hypodermic needle, a butterfly set, or an IV catheter.

The use of hypodermic needles is generally restricted to phlebotomy for obtaining laboratory samples and for single, small injections. As stated in Chapter 7, hypodermic needles are supplied in various diameters (gauges) and lengths. A 2½ inch length is typical for IV needles, and the usual gauges range from 18 to 22 for adults.

A **butterfly set** is preferable to a conventional hypodermic needle for most IV injections and is often used for direct injections with a syringe. This apparatus consists of a needle with plastic projections on either side that aid in holding the needle during venipuncture and that may be taped to the patient's skin after the needle is in place (Fig. 9-1). This prevents movement of the needle in the vein. Attached to the needle is a short length of tubing with a hub that attaches to a syringe. The syringe is filled from a vial or an ampule, and the syringe is then attached to the tubing. Before the butterfly needle is inserted into the vein, the tubing is filled with liquid from the syringe to avoid injecting air into the vein.

IV catheters are frequently used instead of needles or butterfly sets when repeated or continuous IV injections or infusions will be administered. The IV catheter is a two-part system consisting of a needle that fits inside a flexible plastic catheter. The catheter's hub has wing-shaped plastic projections similar to those of the butterfly set. The needle portion is not hollow and serves as a stylet to prevent blood flow through the catheter. This combination unit is inserted into the vein, and the catheter is advanced by slipping it forward over the needle. The catheter is then secured with tape, the needle is withdrawn, and the catheter is connected to the supply system. IV fluid, medication, or ROCM can be administered by syringe through an injection port or IV tubing from a hanging bottle or bag.

An intermittent-injection port (sometimes called a heparin lock) is a small adapter with a diaphragm that is attached to an IV catheter when more than one injection is anticipated.

When a procedure requires the IV infusion of a large volume of fluid, an IV pole and infusion set are needed. Setting up fluid administration equipment is not complicated but is another skill that improves with practice. IV solutions are provided in bottles and plastic bags (Fig. 9-2). The bags have a cap over the sterile port through which the drip chamber of the IV tubing is inserted. The drip chamber is removed from its wrappings and inserted into the sterile port. Care must be taken not to contaminate either component, or both must be discarded.

Solutions supplied in bottles have a removable cap and sometimes a rubber diaphragm covering a rubber stopper. The cap is removed, and the diaphragm is pulled off without touching the stopper. The drip chamber is inserted through the stopper; one must ensure that the clamp on the IV tubing is closed. The bottle or bag may then be inverted and hung on the IV pole. After it is in place, the cover at the other end of the IV tubing is removed, the clamp is opened, and the fluid is allowed to run into a basin until the tubing is free of bubbles. The clamp is then closed and the tip covered to keep it sterile. The procedure is illustrated in Fig. 9-3.

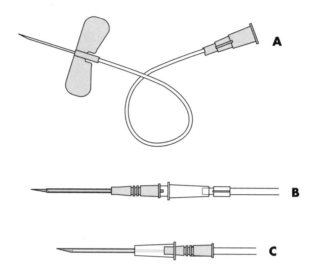

Fig. 9-1   IV needles. **A,** Butterfly needle. **B,** Over-needle catheter. **C,** Through-the-needle catheter.

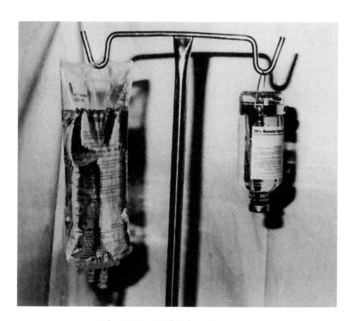

Fig. 9-2   IV fluid packaging.

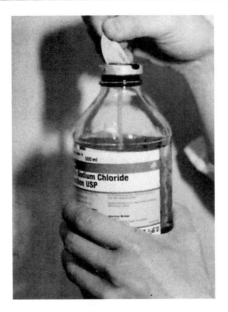

After removing cap, remove diaphragm carefully to avoid contamination.

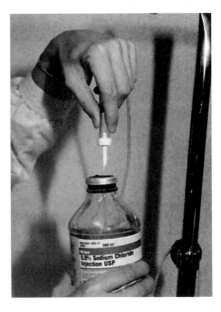

With tubing clamped off, insert drip chamber firmly into access port.

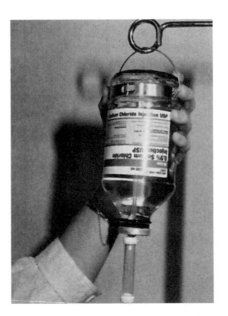

Invert bottle or bag and suspend from pole.

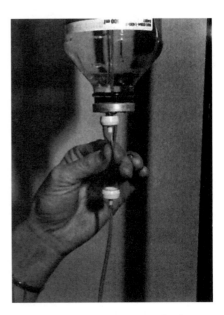

Pinch drip chamber to draw fluid into chamber. Fill chamber about half full.

Fig. 9-3 IV infusion setup.

STARTING AN IV LINE

The veins most often used for initiating IV lines are found in the anterior forearm, the posterior hand, the radial aspect of the wrist, and the **antecubital space** (Fig. 9-4). Usually, the two antecubital veins on each arm are large enough and near enough to the surface to be easily seen. Although they may be the easiest to locate and to puncture, there are drawbacks to their use. Easy access to these veins is important for emer-

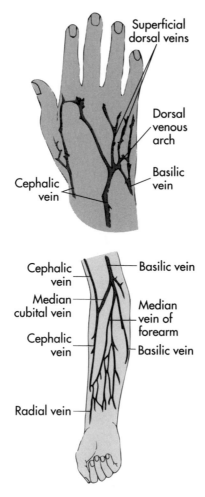

Superficial
dorsal veins

Dorsal
venous
arch

Basilic
vein

Cephalic
vein

Cephalic
vein

Basilic vein

Median
cubital vein

Median
vein of
forearm

Cephalic
vein

Basilic vein

Radial vein

Fig. 9-4 Veins most accessible for venipuncture.

gencies and for routine blood draws. However, overuse may cause these veins to become scarred or sclerotic, which can be a serious problem with patients receiving long-term care. When antecubital IV lines remain in place for some time, they may become uncomfortable and inhibit the patient's ability to flex the elbow. Flexion at the elbow may crimp the catheter, preventing IV flow.

For these reasons, the nursing service tends to use antecubital veins as a last resort. In imaging departments, however, the IV line is usually placed only for the duration of the procedure, and the use of antecubital veins is acceptable when necessary. A vein of adequate size is essential when a bolus of contrast will be delivered at a rapid rate. For small children, this usually requires an antecubital site.

When an IV line is placed in an antecubital vein, a flexible IV catheter should be used. *Never leave a needle in an antecubital vein unless the elbow is restrained in extension by being attached to an armboard.* Flexion of the elbow with a needle in an antecubital vein ruptures the vein, causing extravasation and hematoma.

To select a vein, first secure the tourniquet around the arm above the elbow. Instruct the patient to open and close the hand a few times and then to hold a tight fist. These measures restrict circulation and enlarge the veins, making them easier to identify and to penetrate accurately. The ideal vein can be readily seen and palpated. It is at least twice the diameter of the needle or catheter used, and the vein appears not to bend or curve for a distance at least equal to the length of the needle or catheter. If a suitable vein is not immediately apparent, let the arm hang down for a few seconds; then gently slap the skin over the area where the vein should appear. This may increase the likelihood that the vein will stand out well. If a suitable vein is still not apparent, remove the tourniquet and begin again with the other arm. Fig. 9-5 shows the step-by-step procedure for initiating an IV line using a butterfly setup.

1. Wash your hands.
2. Introduce yourself to the patient, and check the patient's identification band.
3. Address the patient by name, and explain the procedure and the reason it is being done.
4. Ask the patient to remain still during the procedure.
5. Determine the best site for the venipuncture.
6. Cleanse the skin with alcohol or povidone-iodine in a circular motion, starting in the middle and working out to a radius of about 5 cm (2 inches).

8. Verify that you have the proper medication.
9. Put on gloves.
10. Anchor the vein with your nondominant hand or thumb to prevent movement and make the skin taut. This allows easier needle insertion.
11. With the bevel of the needle facing up, puncture the skin at a 20- to 45-degree angle with a quick motion, and insert the needle farther until you feel it pop through the vein. Blood should enter the flash chamber or tubing, indicating that you have entered the vein.

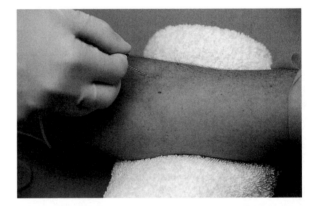

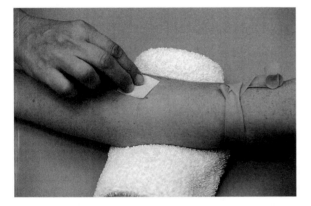

7. Apply a tourniquet 7 to 10 cm (3 to 4 inches) above the site.

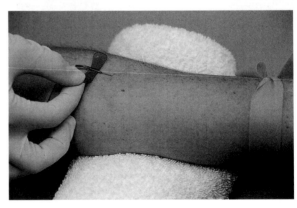

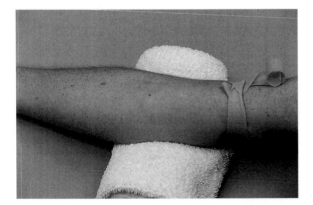

Fig. 9-5 Venipuncture procedure.

12. Decrease the angle of the needle, and insert the needle or catheter ¼ to ½ inch farther into the vein. If you are using an over-the-needle catheter, slowly withdraw the stylet as you insert the catheter. Do not touch the needle or catheter as you insert the needle through the skin; this may allow bacteria to enter the skin with the needle.

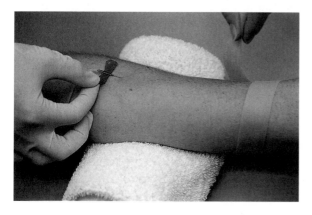

13. Release the tourniquet and attach IV tubing, or if injecting contrast material with a butterfly and syringe, proceed with the injection. Tape the butterfly in place while injecting, to prevent the needle from dislodging.

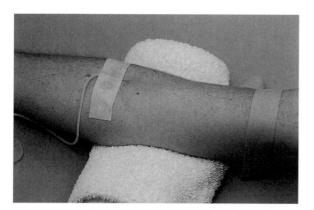

14. *Note:* In some institutions, technologists are taught to perform a ventipuncture as a method for starting an IV drip. In this case, follow your institution's policies for site dressings. Always label the site with the size of needle, the date, and your initials.

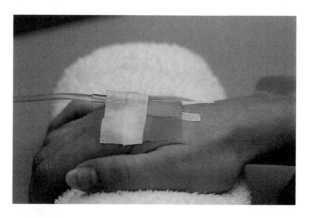

ALERT! If the venipuncture is unsuccessful, withdraw the needle or catheter, and immediately apply light pressure to the insertion site with a cotton ball or gauze. When reattempting a venipuncture, *always* use a new needle.

Fig. 9-5, cont'd For legend see opposite page.

Obese patients may have veins that are too deep to be seen or palpated. Elderly patients may have veins that are easily seen but that may roll under the skin or be too crooked for needle insertion. Patients who have had extensive IV therapy, especially chemotherapy, may have scarred and sclerotic veins that preclude a routine approach. Infants and children also present challenges. Their small veins may be more difficult to see and feel, and the situation is often complicated by the child's refusal or inability to cooperate. Attempt venipuncture only when there is a reasonable expectation of success.

IV MEDICATION ADMINISTRATION

When the IV line has been established, IV medications are typically administered through an intermittent injection port or through access ports on IV infusion tubing. After the patient's identification and the medication label are checked, the correct dose is drawn up into a syringe. The access port is then cleansed with alcohol, and the medication is injected through the port. When an intermittent injection port is used, a small amount of flush solution is injected through the port to prevent blood from coagulating inside the catheter. The system is flushed immediately after it is established, and again after each use, with saline or heparin solution. In many institutions, heparin is used as a flush only with a physician's order.

The hazards posed by needle sticks have prompted the development of "needleless" systems such as the Baxter InterLink IV access system (Fig. 9-6). This system facilitates blood draws and IV medication administration without the use of needles. An important feature of the system is a self-healing rubber substance that is used for medication vial caps, intermittent injection ports, and access ports on IV tubing. These caps and ports can be repeatedly penetrated by blunt plastic cannulas without damaging their integrity. The blunt cannulas are used to draw up medications and to access established IV lines for blood draws and medication administration. The use of a needleless system greatly reduces the incidence of needle use and its attendant hazards in the health care setting.

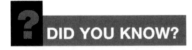
DID YOU KNOW?

The blood urea nitrogen (BUN) and creatinine levels found in a patient's blood are indicators of renal function. Elevated levels of these substances may contraindicate the use of intravascular ROCM, which could cause further stress on renal function. Imaging technologists should check a patient's chart for this information and bring it to the attention of the radiologist prior to administering such contrast media.

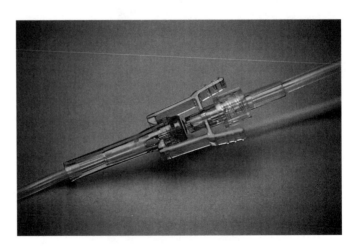

Fig. 9-6 Needleless IV access system.

EXTRAVASATION

Occasionally, IV fluid or medication may accidentally be injected into the tissues surrounding the vein. This **extravasation** (also termed **infiltration**) may be both painful and dangerous. The patient is likely to complain of discomfort, and swelling may be observed at the site. The following precautions are employed to minimize the possibility of extravasation: (1) checking for backflow to determine that the catheter or needle is properly situated before injection, (2) immobilizing the needle or catheter at the injection site, and (3) stopping the injection immediately if the patient complains of discomfort at the injection site or if any resistance to injection is felt.

When extravasation does occur, it is necessary to remove the needle and attend to this problem before proceeding with an injection at another site. Assure the patient that the pain is only temporary. Maintain pressure on the vein until bleeding has stopped completely. This will avoid the additional complication of a **hematoma** at the site of the extravasation. After the bleeding has stopped, the application of hot packs or moist heat to the affected area will help alleviate the pain. It is recommended that an incident report be completed for any extravasation involving a potentially irritating medication or contrast medium. Outpatients should be advised to consult their physicians or to report to the emergency department if inflammation or discomfort persists.

CHARTING MEDICATIONS

When a medication is given by a physician or by a technologist under the physician's supervision, it is always recorded in the patient's chart. The notation is made in the appropriate section of the chart and includes the time of day, the name of the drug, the dose, and the route of administration. A typical entry in the medication record might read: 10:50 AM, Benadryl, 50 mg, PO. Each entry must include the identification of the person who charted it. Initials alone are not considered to be adequate identification. If the medication record calls for initials, there is usually another place in the chart, often on the same page, where each set of initials is identified with the signer's full name (Fig. 9-7). For legal purposes, the technologist who charts medication must use the exact procedure established by the institution.

Any medication prescribed or administered by a physician should be charted by the physician, or it should be countersigned by the physician if it is charted by the technologist. The legal significance of complete accountability in such situations cannot be overemphasized.

The administration of contrast media is sometimes charted as a medication. More often, it is implied by the general charting of the examination and confirmed by a specific statement in the radiologist's report. If the latter method is employed, special notation may be required when there is a variation from the usual medium or dosage for a specific examination.

Although the physician may enter an account of the procedure and medication in the progress notes, the technologist is responsible for

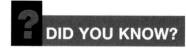

DID YOU KNOW?

Nonionic iodinated contrast media have proved to be less likely to cause an adverse reaction than *ionic* contrast media. Nonionic contrast media do not dissociate into ionic particles when introduced to the bloodstream as do the ionic types of media. This results in a lesser osmotic effect on the cells, which lowers the occurrence of adverse reactions.

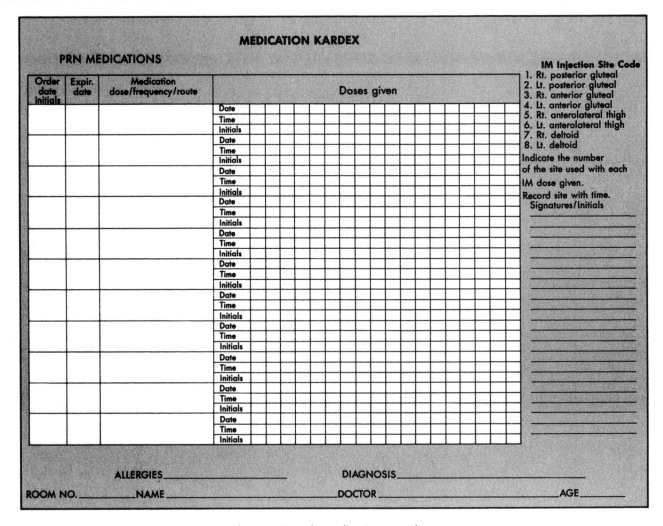

Fig. 9-7 Sample medication record.

checking that the drug, time, dose, and route of administration are clearly delineated for the nursing staff. Charting routines vary widely, so it is best to be familiar with the routine of the specific clinical area.

CONCLUSION

The technologist is called on to play an important role in the administration of medications. Intravenous access systems are used extensively in most hospitals and are the most frequent route of medication administration in imaging departments. The establishment of these systems, as well as their use and monitoring, requires that the technologist have a high degree of knowledge, skill, and awareness.

The charting of medication and the monitoring of patients are significant aspects of medication administration and must not be overlooked. The technologist must recognize the potential harm and legal complications that could result from medication administration errors and strive for error-free performance.

Learning Exercises

True-False Questions

Circle T for true or F for false.

1. **T   F**   The only time a needle may be left in an antecubital vein is when the elbow is restrained in extension by being attached to an armboard.

2. **T   F**   Butterfly sets are used to deliver more than one medication at a time.

3. **T   F**   The drip chamber and port from an IV infusion set are difficult to contaminate.

4. **T   F**   In imaging departments IV lines are usually placed only for the duration of the procedure; therefore, use of antecubital veins is acceptable.

5. **T   F**   Elevated levels of blood urea nitrogen and creatinine in a patient's blood may contraindicate the use of intravascular ROCM.

6. **T   F**   Ionic contrast media are less likely to cause an adverse reaction.

7. **T   F**   The veins most often used for initiating IV lines are found in the anterior forearm, the posterior hand, the radial aspect of the wrist, and the antecubital space.

Fill-in-the-Blank Questions

1. _____ is the accidental injection of IV fluid or medication into the tissues surrounding the vein.

2. The area in front of the elbow (the bend) is known as _____,

3. A(n) _____ is a collection of blood in the tissues of the skin or an organ.

4. A(n) _____ (sometimes called a heparin lock) is a small adapter with a diaphragm that is attached to an IV catheter when more than one injection is anticipated.

5. Checking for backflow, immobilizing the needle at the injection site, and stopping the injection immediately if the patient complains of discomfort are three ways to minimize the possibility of _____.

6. _____ patients may have veins that are too deep to be seen or palpated; _____ patients may have veins that are easily seen but that may roll under the skin.

7. The two most common replacement fluids for dehydrated patients are _____ and a 5% solution of _____.

Review Questions

1. What steps may be taken to adequately locate an acceptable vein for venipuncture?

2. What should be done if an ROCM infiltrates the tissues?

3. When an immediate response to a medication is critical, how should the drug be delivered?

4. What precautions should be taken when disposing of used syringes and needles?

5. What information should be placed in the patient's chart following administration of ROCM?

Pharmacology of Emergency Medications

10

OBJECTIVES

At the conclusion of this chapter you should be able to:
1. Define cardiac arrest and respiratory arrest.
2. State the basic steps involved in managing a patient in cardiac arrest in the radiology department.
3. Define CPR, ACLS, BLS, and Code Blue.
4. Identify the most commonly used emergency medications for cardiac arrest.
5. Describe the coloration of outdated cardiac drugs found in the drug box or cart.

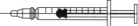

KEY TERMS

metabolic acidosis
advanced cardiac life support (ACLS)
alpha receptors
antidiuretic hormone (ADH)
atropine
basic life support (BLS)
beta receptors
cardiac arrest
cardiopulmonary resuscitation (CPR)
Code Blue
dopamine
epinephrine
lidocaine
muscarinic receptor
normal sinus rhythm (NSR)
premature ventricular contractions (PVCs)
respiratory arrest
return of spontaneous circulation (ROSC)
sodium bicarbonate
ventricular fibrillation

INTRODUCTION

Patients are frequently transported to the radiology department under the direct care and supervision of the imaging technologist. Eventually, the technologist will have to deal with a patient suffering an acute life-threatening condition requiring emergency action. Therefore, these professionals should have a basic understanding of life-threatening emergencies that can occur in the radiology suite. Since this book deals primarily with pharmacology, emergency conditions not treated by drug intervention, such as choking, seizures, fainting, shock, and diabetic emergencies, will not be discussed. These conditions may be life threatening, and the technologist should be skilled in recognizing and providing treatment. The most common emergency in the radiology department requiring drug therapy is cardiorespiratory arrest. This condition and the drugs used to treat it will be discussed in detail.

CARDIORESPIRATORY ARREST

Cardiac arrest is a condition wherein the heart ceases to adequately pump blood to the rest of the body. A **respiratory arrest** is a condition wherein the patient becomes unable to breathe; thus the body is inadequately oxygenated. If not treated promptly, a respiratory arrest will progress to a full cardiac arrest (known as cardiorespiratory arrest). A full cardiac arrest becomes lethal if immediate intervention does not occur. Management of cardiac arrest requires a systematic approach.

The American Heart Association states that the highest survival rate following cardiac arrest occurs in patients who receive **cardiopulmonary resuscitation (CPR)** within four minutes and who are additionally provided medications via **advanced cardiac life support (ACLS)** within eight minutes. *Time is life!* The patient with no blood circulation for more than four minutes will likely suffer brain damage. If spontaneous circulation is not restored within eight minutes, the patient will probably die. It is for these reasons that the technologist cannot solely rely on other medical professionals to provide care to patients suffering a life-threatening emergent condition. A medical imaging technologist can call for help and then begin **basic life support (BLS),** as outlined by the American Heart Association or American Red Cross, until assistance arrives. Every technologist should be certified in basic life support. However, prudence would dictate the technologist be prepared for the possibility that the emergency team may be delayed or need extra assistance. Therefore, familiarity with advanced life support procedures and medications is recommended.

ACLS is a set of guidelines developed by the American Heart Association (AHA) for use in managing a patient undergoing cardiac arrest. Specific treatment methods are outlined in the ACLS guidelines and can be utilized for treating victims of cardiac arrest. These protocols are especially helpful for health care professionals who are occasionally confronted with a cardiac arrest patient. When a clinical dilemma of this magnitude and urgency occurs, inexperienced personnel require guidelines or protocols that can be quickly and easily consulted so that the correct treatment steps can be initiated.

The technologist should also be familiar with emergency pager systems so that emergency assistance can be summoned swiftly and efficiently. Generally, a standardized phrase such as **Code Blue** or a fictitious doctor's name such as "Dr. Stat" is used to summon an emergency team to the area requiring immediate assistance. Each medical facility has its own procedure to call for emergency assistance. It is the professional duty of the medical imaging technologist to know this procedure clearly.

EMERGENCY MEDICATIONS FOR CARDIORESPIRATORY ARREST

Preparation made in advance of any emergency is critical. In addition to life support skill, personnel should be familiar with the emergency medication box or cart. See Fig. 10-1.

The technologist should check the emergency medication box (or cart) at least monthly to ensure that all drugs are present, in adequate supply, and have not expired. The box should also be checked and restocked after each emergency use. Medical imaging technologists should become familiar with the contents, drug names, location within the box, proper use, and pharmacology. Acquiring this knowledge and expertise allows the technologist to accurately predict which drug will most likely be needed and thus rapidly acquire it for the emergency team. This makes for swift and efficient handling of emergency situations.

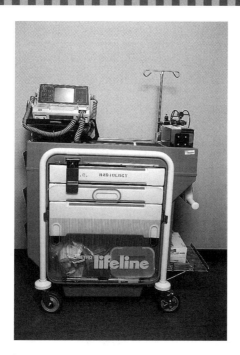

Fig. 10-1 Emergency cart with defibrillator.

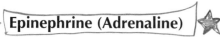

Epinephrine (Adrenaline)

Epinephrine is currently one of the most valuable, potentially lifesaving therapeutic agents available to cardiac arrest victims. This drug is the pharmaceutical equivalent of adrenaline, produced by the adrenal gland.

Pharmacodynamics. Epinephrine elicits sympathomimetic (mimics the sympathetic nervous system) effects on various organ systems by attaching to and stimulating the $alpha_1$, $alpha_2$, $beta_1$, and/or $beta_2$ receptors. Table 10-1 outlines the various effects that can occur when these receptors are stimulated by epinephrine. The effects of epinephrine on the various receptors are dose dependent. Low doses generally result in **beta receptor** predominance, whereas higher doses result in **alpha receptor** predominance. In cardiac arrest, epinephrine is primarily given in doses sufficient to stimulate $alpha_1$ receptors so that arterioles (small blood vessels) can constrict. This produces a marked increase in blood pressure. When combined with chest compressions, epinephrine will hopefully cause a **return of spontaneous circulation (ROSC).**

Although it is thought that $beta_1$ receptors play no role in ROSC, epinephrine stimulation of these receptors in various organ systems may contribute to increasing and sustaining blood pressure. In the myocardium, $beta_1$ receptor stimulation leads to increased force of contraction, rate, and cardiac output. $Beta_1$ receptor stimulation in the kidneys causes release of a hormone called renin, which eventually helps produce a potent vasoconstrictive substance in the blood known as angiotensin II. Angiotensin II in turn stimulates the adrenal gland to secrete

Adrenalin/
Epinephrin is a
- vasoconstrictor (vessels contract)
- bronch dialator (airway open)
- ↑ BP - contracts skeletal muscles
- ↑ HR
- ↑ CO - ↓ diuresis
(body ↓ urine: keeps urine in)

used for Cardiac Arrests
bronchospasms
anaphylaxis (allergic reaction)

Table 10-1 Pharmacodynamic Effects of the Adrenergic Receptors*

alpha$_1$	Increases blood pressure, dilates pupils, decreases ability to urinate and defecate
alpha$_2$	Decreases blood pressure (when stimulated in the brain), causes constipation
beta$_1$	Increases heart rate, cardiac output, and dysrhythmias; causes fat to break down (lipolysis); releases renin hormone from the kidneys (may lead to increased blood pressure)
beta$_2$	Decreases blood pressure, opens airways, causes constipation, inhibits uterine contractions, increases glucose production, releases insulin, contracts skeletal muscle
dopamine	Vasodilation of renal, coronary, intracerebral, and mesenteric blood vessels

*The effects listed are seen when the receptor is stimulated; if more than one receptor is stimulated at any given moment, the effects seen may be mixed.

a hormone called aldosterone, which travels to the kidneys, where it acts to facilitate salt and water retention. The process is collectively known as the renin-angiotensin-aldosterone system and ultimately leads to increased blood pressure when activated.

Epinephrine also stimulates beta$_1$ receptors in the posterior pituitary gland (located at the base of the brain) to cause release of **antidiuretic hormone (ADH,** vasopressin), which is also a potent vasoconstrictor and water preserver. Again, the combination of vasoconstriction and water preservation leads to an increase in blood pressure.

Pharmacokinetics. Epinephrine has an onset of action of approximately 1 to 2 minutes, with a duration of action of approximately 2 to 10 minutes. Once inside tissues, epinephrine is rapidly metabolized and inactivated by the enzymes catechol-*O*-methyltransferase (COMT) and monoamine oxidase (MAO). The resulting sulfate and glucuronide metabolites of epinephrine are excreted in the urine.

Indications. Epinephrine is indicated first line for cardiorespiratory arrest and is used as such in **ventricular fibrillation,** asystole, and electromechanical dissociation (EMD). Other uses include treatment of anaphylactic or anaphylactoid reactions and acute bronchospasm. Table 10-2 lists the available epinephrine preparations used for cardiac arrest.

Dosage and administration. Conventional ACLS guidelines recommend epinephrine 0.5 to 1.0 mg (0.01 to 0.015 mg/kg) every 5 to 10 minutes as needed to attain return of spontaneous circulation. Five to 10 ml of a 1:10,000 solution is equivalent to 0.5 to 1.0 mg. Some medication carts will carry a 30-ml vial of a 1:1000 ml solution, which is equivalent to 1 mg/ml. In the pediatric patient, 0.01 mg/kg to 0.015 mg/kg should be used.

The dosage range for epinephrine has recently been scrutinized, and has been considered by many to be ineffectively low. The AHA has

Table 10-2   Common Parenteral Forms of Emergency Medications

Drug	Route*	Concentration	Volume
Epinephrine	IM, IV, SC, ET, IO	1.0 mg/ml (1:1000)	1 ml ampule
		1.0 mg/ml (1:1000)	1 ml vial
		1.0 mg/ml (1:1000)	30 ml vial
		0.1 mg/ml (1:10,000)	10 ml syringe
		0.01 mg/ml (1:100,000)[†]	5 ml syringe
Dopamine	IV	0.8 mg/ml (800 μg/ml)	250 and 500 ml bag
		1.6 mg/ml (1600 μg/ml)	250 and 500 ml bag
		40 mg/ml (40,000 μg/ml)	5, 10, 20 ml vial
		80 mg/ml (80,000 μg/ml)	5, 20 ml vials
		80 mg/ml (80,000 μg/ml)	10 ml syringe
		160 mg/ml (160,000 μg/ml)	5 ml vials
Atropine	IV, ET, IO	0.05 mg/ml	5 ml syringe
		0.10 mg/ml	10 ml syringe
		0.30 mg/ml	1, 30 ml vial
		0.40 mg/ml	1, 20, 30 ml vial
		0.50 mg/ml	5 ml syringe
		0.80 mg/ml	0.5 ml syringe
		1.0 mg/ml	10 ml syringe
Lidocaine (for direct IV administration)	IV, ET, IO	10 mg/ml	5 ml syringe
		10 mg/ml	20, 30, 50 ml vial
		20 mg/ml	5 ml syringe
Lidocaine (for IV admixture)	IV	40 mg/ml	25, 50 ml vials
		40 mg/ml	25, 50 ml syringe
		100 mg/ml	10 ml vial
		200 mg/ml	10 ml vial
Lidocaine in D_5W (premixed IV infusion)	IV	2 mg/ml	500, 1000 ml bag
		4 mg/ml	250, 500 ml bag
		8 mg/ml	250, 500 ml bag
Sodium bicarbonate	IV, IO	0.5 mEq/ml	5, 10 ml syringe
		0.9 mEq/ml	50 ml syringe
		1.0 mEq/ml	10, 50 ml syringe

*ET = endotracheal; IO = intraosseous (generally used in pediatrics).
[†]1:100,000 concentration; 5 ml syringe is a pediatric formulation.

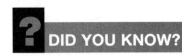

since revised its guidelines to include adult epinephrine doses greater than 1 mg after the first round of medication fails to attain ROSC. Doses greater than 1.0 mg are considered "high dose." Both recent research and old research suggest that doses as high as 15 mg may be required to attain ROSC in some adult individuals. The technologist is encouraged to keep up with the current literature on this controversial subject, as doses may change from one year to the next.

Epinephrine may be administered intravenously through a peripheral or central vein, down the endotracheal tube (intrapulmonary administration), intraosseously (into the bone lumen) in pediatrics, or via intracardiac injection into the left ventricle; please note that intracardiac injection is not widely practiced at this time, since myocardial necrosis can occur secondarily. The intraosseous and endotracheal routes are important to keep in mind; many practitioners forget about these routes in the excitement of an actual emergency. Intraosseous injection is very effective in pediatric patients. Endotracheal administration is very effective in both pediatric and adult patients.

Endotracheal administration is generally performed when no intravenous access is available. To perform this technique, the medication should be diluted to a total volume of 10 ml, squirted down the endotracheal tube, and then followed by at least three rapid ventilations via bag-valve mask. These rapid ventilations serve to disperse the medication over the large surface area of the lung so that systemic absorption can take place. This technique has been documented to be effective at delivering epinephrine to the systemic circulation during cardiac arrest.

Adverse effects. Major adverse effects seen with epinephrine consist of cardiac dysrhythmias, including ventricular fibrillation, via beta$_1$ receptor stimulation in the heart. Epinephrine may also lead to increased ischemia in an already damaged heart, as the oxygen demand exceeds the oxygen supply in cardiorespiratory arrest. However, in cardiac arrest the benefits generally outweigh the risks. If the patient survives the cardiac arrest, then hypertension and dysrhythmias should be expected. Other major adverse effects include a sense of nervousness, headache, and muscle twitching (fasciculations).

Stability. Epinephrine products are unstable when exposed to light for long periods of time and may turn pink or brown. Discolored solutions should not be used, as they may be ineffective. Checking your medication stock frequently can help to avoid this problem.

Dopamine (Intropin)

Dopamine is the pharmaceutical equivalent of endogenous dopamine. Endogenous dopamine is a precursor to norepinephrine and epinephrine naturally produced by the body.

Pharmacodynamics. Dopamine has dose-dependent effects on the various sympathetic (adrenergic) nervous system receptors. At low doses, dopamine primarily stimulates the dopamine receptors in the renal, coronary, intracerebral, and mesenteric arteries. This leads to arteriolar vasodilation with increased blood flow to the respective organs. At moderate doses, dopamine will also begin stimulating the $beta_1$ receptors to cause increases in contractility, force of contraction, and stroke volume in the myocardium. This effectively increases cardiac output in patients suffering shock and/or congestive heart failure. At high doses, dopamine begins stimulating alpha receptors. When high doses are used, the net effects are a combination of dopamine, $beta_1$, $alpha_1$, and $alpha_2$ receptor stimulation. No $beta_2$ receptor stimulation occurs. At very high doses, the primary pharmacodynamic effects seen are those associated with $alpha_1$ receptor stimulation.

Pharmacokinetics. Dopamine has an onset of action of approximately 2 to 4 minutes, with a duration of action of less than 10 minutes. Renal vasodilation with increased urine output may take up to 20 minutes. Dopamine is metabolized to homovallinic acid (HVA), norepinephrine, and other chemicals by the enzymes catechol-*O*-methyltransferase and monamine oxidase. The resulting metabolites of dopamine are excreted in the urine. A small fraction of dopamine is excreted unchanged in the urine.

Indications. Dopamine is indicated for treating hypotension secondary to congestive heart failure, myocardial infarction, trauma, sepsis, and overt heart failure. Dopamine is also used to increase urine output in patients suffering renal failure. In cardiac arrest, dopamine is used second line, after epinephrine and fluids have failed to attain ROSC. Dopamine is also used to further support blood pressure following successful ROSC in cardiac arrest victims.

Dosage and administration. Dopamine is administered by intravenous infusion via a controlled delivery device such as an electronic pump. The appropriate total dose should be diluted in either normal saline (NS) or 5% dextrose in water (D_5W). Low-dose dopamine is considered to be less than 5 $\mu g/kg/min$. Intermediate dosing is between 5 and 10 $\mu g/kg/min$. High-dose dopamine is generally considered to be any dose above 10 $\mu g/kg/min$.

Generally, dopamine is used as the premixed solution. Table 10-2 lists available dopamine preparations. If mixing the solution is required, then an easy method is by placing 800 mg into 500 ml of either D_5W or NS and attaching a microdrip (60 drops/ml calibration) tubing set to the infusion bag. This gives a total concentration of 1600 $\mu g/ml$. An average 70-kg patient would then require approximately 700 $\mu g/min$ (10 $\mu g/kg/min$) for $alpha_1$ receptor effects to increase blood pressure. This calculates to be 42,000 $\mu g/hr$ (700 $\mu g/min$ × 60 min), which is approximately 26 ml/hr of the 1600 $\mu g/ml$ solution. By using the microdrip tubing, the technologist can easily titrate the drip rate to 26 drops/min, which is equal to 26 ml/hr. (NOTE: if macrodrip tubing [calibrated at 15 drops/ml] is used, then the drip rate per minute is equal to ml/hr divided by 4; approximately 6.5 drops/min = 26 ml/hr.)

Adverse effects. Dopamine produces dose-dependent adverse effects. Hypotension occurs with low doses. Hypertension, cardiac dysrhythmias, headache, nausea, vomiting, angina pectoris, and/or tachycardia may occur with high doses. If dopamine extravasates into surrounding tissues, then necrosis may occur. Gangrene of the extremities has occurred with high-dose infusions in patients with diabetes or vascular occlusive diseases. Phenytoin (Dilantin) may interact with dopamine and cause hypotension, bradycardia, and/or seizures.

Stability. Dopamine is generally stable for up to 24 hours when placed into solution. Commercially prepared solutions are stable until the expiration date listed on the product. Dopamine products are unstable when exposed to light for long periods of time and should be protected from light when in storage. Discolored solutions should not be used, as they may be ineffective. Checking the medication stock frequently can help to avoid this problem. Dopamine is incompatible with sodium bicarbonate, iron salts, and oxidizing agents.

Atropine

Atropine is an antimuscarinic agent frequently used in patients suffering from cardiac arrest.

Pharmacodynamics. Atropine competitively inhibits the action of acetylcholine or other cholinergic stimuli at the **muscarinic receptors** in the parasympathetic nervous system. Table 10-3 lists the various effects that occur when muscarinic receptors are *stimulated* in the parasympathetic nervous system; the competitive inhibition of these receptors by atropine generally yields the *opposite effect.*

Atropine is used in the setting of cardiac arrest when a patient exhibits bradycardia (slow heart rate) on the cardiac monitor. When the heart rate falls to 40 beats/min or less, the emergency medical team will use atropine to competitively block the muscarinic receptors in the myocardium. This blunts the effects of the parasympathetic nervous system on the heart while allowing the sympathetic nervous system to function unopposed; keep in mind that the parasympathetic nervous system and the sympathetic nervous system generally counter-regulate each other in almost all tissues and organs. The sympathetic nervous system will thus stimulate the beta$_1$ receptors with the neurotransmitter norepinephrine, resulting in increased heart rate, contractility, and conduction velocity. In addition, if epinephrine or dopamine is currently in use, then their actions on the beta$_1$ receptors of the heart will be enhanced following atropine administration.

Pharmacokinetics. Atropine has an onset of action of approximately 2 to 4 minutes following intravenous administration. Atropine is absorbed via the oral, intramuscular, and pulmonary routes; however, the intravenous and endotracheal (pulmonary) routes are the only accepted routes for cardiac arrest victims. Atropine distributes well

Table 10-3   Effects of Muscarinic (Cholinergic) Receptors When Stimulated*

Pupillary constriction (miosis)
Decreased heart rate (bradycardia)
Decreased heart conduction velocity
Decreased heart contractility
Arteriolar vasodilation
Bronchial smooth muscle contraction
Bronchial gland secretions
Gastrointestinal peristalsis
Gastrointestinal secretions
Gastrointestinal sphincter relaxation
Salivation
Urinary bladder contraction
Urinary sphincter relaxation
Sweat gland secretion
Glycogen synthesis

*Atropine generally blocks these effects and may lead to the opposite reactions.

throughout the body and will lead to side effects in the parasympathetic nervous system. Atropine is metabolized by the liver to tropic acid, tropine, tropic acid esters, and glucuronide conjugates. The half-life of elimination for atropine is approximately 2 to 3 hours. Atropine and its metabolites are eliminated principally in the urine, yet some may be excreted via pulmonary exhalation.

Indications. Atropine is indicated for cardiac arrest patients who are suffering hemodynamically significant bradycardia, first-degree atrioventricular block, and/or ventricular asystole (flatline). Atropine may also be used when attempts at intubation lead to vagal nerve (a parasympathetic nerve) stimulation resulting in symptomatic bradycardia.

Dosage and administration. Atropine should be given via rapid intravenous push at doses ranging from 0.5 to 1.0 mg every 3 to 5 minutes until the desired heart rate is achieved. Ventricular asystole generally requires at least 1.0 mg. A cumulative dose of 3.0 mg generally should not be exceeded, as this will lead to complete vagus nerve blockade. Pediatric patients require 0.02 mg/kg, with a minimum dose of 0.1 mg and a maximum single dose of 0.5 mg in children and 1.0 mg in adolescents, respectively; the cumulative maximum dose for children is 1.0 mg and for adolescents 2.0 mg.

If atropine is given via slow intravenous push, a paradoxical action may occur leading to a further decrease in heart rate that could be lethal. If the intravenous route is unavailable, then either the endotracheal or the intraosseous route can be used. The technique for endotracheal administration is the same as that for epinephrine discussed previously.

Adverse effects. Serious adverse effects of atropine include a worsening of myocardial ischemia or extension of infarct zone, ventricular fibrillation, and ventricular tachycardia. A paradoxical

Lidocaine- has an affect
on electrical impulses
of ♡ ∴ making more
reg. – used w/ ventricular
fibulation (flutters ⇒ different
parts of ventrical flutter
once.)

slowing of heart rate may occur with low doses of atropine or in patients who receive the drug via slow intravenous push. Less severe adverse effects include dry mouth, blurred vision, constipation, urinary retention, pupillary dilation (mydriasis), headache, nervousness, progression of angle-closure glaucoma, drowsiness, weakness, dizziness, flushing, insomnia, nausea, vomiting, gastrointestinal bloating, bad taste in mouth, mental confusion, and central nervous system excitement.

Stability. Commercially prepared atropine injections are stable until the expiration date listed on the product. Atropine products are unstable when exposed to light for long periods of time and should be protected from light when in storage. Atropine is incompatible with sodium bicarbonate, norepinephrine, metaraminol bitartrate, methohexitol, and pentobarbital.

Lidocaine (Xylocaine)

Lidocaine is one of the most frequently used antidysrhythmic (antiarrhythmic) drugs for patients suffering from cardiac arrest.

Pharmacodynamics. The myocardium has an extensive electrical conduction system that works in coordination with the parasympathetic and sympathetic nervous systems. Chemical electrolytes such as sodium, calcium, magnesium, and potassium play an integral role in the electrical activity of the conduction system of the heart. An improper balance of these electrolytes can lead to life-threatening cardiac dysrhythmias. Lidocaine is an antidysrhythmic agent that pharmacologically blocks sodium channels, thus blocking sodium electrolyte, which affects the myocardial ventricles. This mechanism of action allows lidocaine to effectively terminate **premature ventricular contractions (PVCs)** and/or convert a ventricular tachycardia to a slower, more stable cardiac rhythm such as **normal sinus rhythm (NSR).** If multiple PVCs and/or ventricular tachycardia were allowed to continue in the cardiac arrest patient, then a severe decrease in cardiac output could lead to the patient's death.

Pharmacokinetics. Lidocaine has an onset of action of approximately 30 to 90 seconds following intravenous administration and 10 minutes following intramuscular administration. Lidocaine reaches significant serum levels only when absorbed via the intravenous, intramuscular, and pulmonary routes. This drug distributes rapidly out of the bloodstream and into tissues throughout the body following intravenous administration. Lidocaine requires a steady serum concentration between 1.5 and 6.0 μg/ml to maintain therapeutic action. For this reason and because of its rapid distribution out of the bloodstream into tissues, lidocaine usually requires two bolus doses approximately 10 minutes apart initially, followed by a continuous intravenous drip to maintain its serum concentration in the therapeutic range. It is metabolized by the liver to monoethylglycinexylidide (MEGX)

❓ DID YOU KNOW?

Before beginning invasive procedures or injecting patients with contrast agents, you should obtain a thorough medical history, including information about any existing cardiac arrhythmias, and assess baseline vital signs. An irregular cardiac rhythm in a patient with a cardiovascular disease such as coronary artery disease or who has had a myocardial infarction or open-heart surgery can quickly progress to a cardiac arrest.

and glycinexylidide (GX). These metabolites are active in producing pharmacologic effects. Lidocaine has a half-life of elimination of approximately 80 to 108 minutes in normal individuals, but this may be as long as 7 hours in patients with heart failure. Lidocaine and its metabolites are eliminated primarily by the kidneys.

Indications. Lidocaine is indicated for treating ventricular dysrhythmias in heart attack or cardiac arrest. Following cardiac arrest, lidocaine is primarily used to treat ventricular tachycardia. It can be used to treat ventricular fibrillation when direct-current electrical shock (i.e., defibrillation) has failed. If defibrillation is successful in converting the heart rhythm to normal sinus rhythm, lidocaine should be used as a follow-up to stabilize the heart.

Dosage and administration. Lidocaine is administered as an initial IV bolus dose of 1.0 mg/kg body weight (the usual adult dose is 50 to 100 mg) and repeated every 5 to 10 minutes as needed to suppress ventricular dysrhythmias. The total, cumulative bolus dose should not exceed 3 mg/kg. Patients with congestive heart failure should receive only 50% of the total dose to avoid toxicity. Lidocaine is available in a prepared syringe for emergency use (Table 10-2). (Lidocaine can also be effectively administered via the endotracheal tube and the intraosseous route; the techniques are the same as for epinephrine.)

Immediately after the first bolus dose, an intravenous lidocaine drip at the rate of 2 mg/min should be started; in pediatrics, the infusion rate should be 20 μg/kg/min. Patients with congestive heart failure should receive only 50% of the total dose to avoid toxicity. A lidocaine infusion can be prepared by adding 1 g (1000 mg) of lidocaine to 250 ml NS or D_5W for a concentration of 4 mg/ml; the IV pump rate then required to give a 2 mg/min infusion is 30 ml/hr; for pediatrics. dosage calculation should be based on 20 μg/kg/min. Table 10-2 lists other lidocaine preparations that can be used.

Adverse effects. Adverse effects of lidocaine usually occur when it is infused too rapidly to a conscious patient, when excessive doses are used, or when a drug-drug interaction occurs. Mild lidocaine toxicity includes drowsiness, confusion, nausea, dizziness, gait disturbances (ataxia), ringing in the ears (tinnitus), numbness (paresthesias), and muscle twitching (fasciculations). Severe toxicity includes psychosis, seizures, and respiratory depression.

Stability. Commercially prepared lidocaine injections are stable until the expiration date listed on the product. Lidocaine products are unstable when exposed to excessive heat (greater than 40° C). Preparations made by adding lidocaine to D_5W or NS are stable for 24 hours at room temperature. Lidocaine may adversely affect the action of dopamine, epinephrine, norepinephrine, and isoproterenol. It is best to administer lidocaine through a separate IV line, if possible.

Sodium Bicarbonate

Sodium bicarbonate is a strong alkalinizing agent. Its use for treating cardiac arrest has been seriously scrutinized in the recent past. However, it is still frequently utilized in select patients as described below.

Pharmacodynamics. Sodium bicarbonate is an alkalinizing agent that dissociates into its chemical components to liberate bicarbonate ion (HCO_3^-). The human body has many chemical buffers to maintain the acid-base homeostasis of its tissues. Bicarbonate serves as a principal component of one of the main buffer systems, known as the *bicarbonate–carbonic acid buffer.* The pulmonary and renal systems are major contributors to this system. The following is a very simplistic description of how the bicarbonate–carbonic acid buffer system functions on a clinical basis in the event of cardiac arrest–induced acidosis; the student is referred to advanced literature for a more complete understanding of physiologic buffer systems.

If the body is producing too much acid via metabolic processes (i.e., metabolic acidosis), then the lungs will increase carbonic acid (CO_2) excretion via increased respiratory rate in patients who are capable of breathing; carbonic acid is excreted into the atmosphere by the lungs. The kidney will also retain HCO_3^- to help buffer the acid produced. These two mechanisms effectively maintain the acid-base balance of the body. If the patient is incapable of breathing rapidly enough or the amount of HCO_3^- is significantly depleted, then excessive acid may increase in the body and lead to clinical acidosis, which can be severely detrimental to health.

During cardiorespiratory arrest, the patient generally cannot adequately ventilate. The body then begins a process of respiration known as anaerobic (without oxygen) respiration to help supply energy to tissues. Anaerobic respiration is a very ineffective way of supplying food to tissues. The end product of anaerobic respiration is *lactic acid.* When lactic acid accumulates to critical levels, the body suffers from extreme **metabolic acidosis.** This can be lethal in cardiorespiratory arrest patients. A combination of sodium bicarbonate and artificial respiration is used to combat severe acidosis in cardiorespiratory arrest. Intravenously administered sodium bicarbonate is used in hopes of restoring HCO_3^- body stores depleted during the clinical deterioration of the patient.

Note of interest: It is quite possible that administering sodium bicarbonate to a severely acidotic patient may actually make the tissue acidosis worse and thus be more detrimental to the patient. This paradox may occur because during the metabolism of sodium bicarbonate a CO_2 molecule (an acidic compound) is liberated as well as an HCO_3^- ion; the CO_2 molecule may distribute more rapidly into tissue than the HCO_3^- ion, thus producing a severe acidosis prior to the $HCO_3^-:CO_2:H^+$ equilibrium. For this reason, sodium bicarbonate is no longer recommended as an absolute. It is recommended to be used *only* if the physician deems it necessary based on clinical factors taken into consideration.

Pharmacokinetics. Specific pharmacokinetic data are not relevant to the use of sodium bicarbonate in cardiac arrest patients. Determination of bicarbonate need is guided by serum pH, HCO_3^-, and P_{CO_2}. These are expressed chemically in the body by the chemical equation known as the Henderson-Hasselbach equation:

$$pH = 6.1 + \log \frac{[HCO_3^-]}{0.03 \times P_{CO_2}}$$

where:

$$pH = \text{potential of hydrogen ion} = \log \frac{1}{H^+}$$

$$6.1 = \text{a constant}$$
$$[HCO_3^-] = \text{concentration of bicarbonate in mEq/L}$$

Indications. Sodium bicarbonate may be used for treating severe metabolic or respiratory acidosis.

Dosage and administration. Sodium bicarbonate is usually administered via rapid IV infusion push during cardiac arrest. In pediatric cardiac arrest, this medication can be delivered via intraosseous injection. In adult cardiac arrest patients, 1 mEq/kg may be given initially, followed by 0.5 mEq/kg every 10 minutes during continued arrest. Adequate ventilation must be performed in addition to sodium bicarbonate, since ventilation is an important mechanism for correcting severe metabolic acidosis. Children should receive the pediatric formula at an initial dose of 1 mEq/kg via *slow* IV push. Using the adult formulation or rapid IV push in small children or neonates can lead to hypertonicity because of the high sodium concentration. If arterial blood gas values are available, then the dose of sodium bicarbonate should be calculated via the following formula:

$$\text{Sodium bicarbonate (mEq)} = 0.3 \times \text{Body weight (in kg)} \times \text{Base deficit}$$

Base deficit is equal to the normal serum HCO_3^- minus the measured serum HCO_3^-.

Adverse effects. Extravasation of IV sodium bicarbonate can lead to cellulitis, tissue necrosis, ulceration, and/or sloughing. Metabolic alkalosis can occur with excessive doses or in patients with renal dysfunction. Metabolic alkalosis can cause ionized calcium to decrease, resulting in irritability and muscle tetany. Metabolic alkalosis may also decrease oxygen release from hemoglobin, thus resulting in tissue hypoxia, anaerobic respiration, and lactic acid production. The high sodium content of this medication can lead to osmotic fluid shifts with resultant increases in intravascular fluid. Congestive heart failure may then occur. Finally, serum potassium concentrations may decrease via ion shift during sodium bicarbonate therapy.

Stability. Commercially prepared sodium bicarbonate injections are stable until the expiration date listed on the product. Sodium bicarbonate injection is stable at temperatures ranging from 15° to 30° C. This medication is incompatible with many medications, including calcium salts, epinephrine, dopamine, and lidocaine. Either a separate IV line should be used or the line should be flushed with normal saline prior to sodium bicarbonate injection.

OTHER CARDIAC EMERGENCY MEDICATIONS

This chapter is intended to describe medications that are generally used first line for treating cardiorespiratory arrest. The student is encouraged to use one of the reference books mentioned in Chapter 2 to look up and learn about other potential drugs of use, including procainamide, bretylium, amiodarone, digoxin, adenosine, magnesium, calcium, isoproterenol, verapamil, diltiazem, metoprolol, propranolol, labetalol, norepinephrine, dobutamine, amrinone, milrinone, nitroglycerin, and nitroprusside.

CONCLUSION

Cardiorespiratory arrest is a clinical dilemma that all medical professionals who work in or around a hospital setting will eventually be confronted with. Even those who work in the clinic setting may see this life-threatening situation. Death usually ensues if medications are not administered within the first eight minutes of arrest. It is obvious that all medical professionals should become familiar with at least the treatment that is initially required to save a patient's life. This chapter is designed to give the imaging technologist a good overview of the major medications used in the first few minutes of cardiorespiratory arrest. By understanding the pharmacologic principles behind the medications, the radiologic technologist can at least summon help and have the medication cart out, open, and ready for use by the emergency team. This may be one of the most important functions you ever perform for your patient. Understanding the concepts presented in this chapter could be the difference between life and death for your patient! After all, what good is the radiologic diagnosis if the patient dies prior to treatment?

Learning Exercises

Abbreviations
Spell out each of the abbreviations below.

1. ACLS: *Advanced Cardiac Life Support*

2. ADH: *Antidiretic Hormone*

3. BLS: *Basic Life Support*

4. AHA: *Am. Heart Assoc.*

5. CPR: *Cardio Pulmon resescitation*

True-False
Circle T for true or F for false.

1. **(T)** F Cardiac arrest is a condition wherein the heart ceases to adequately pump blood to the rest of the body.

2. **(T)** F ACLS is a set of guidelines developed by the AHA for use in managing the patient undergoing cardiopulmonary arrest.

3. T **(F)** Technologists should check the emergency medication box at least twice a year to ensure that all drugs are present, in adequate supply, and have not expired.

4. **(T)** F When combined with chest compressions, epinephrine will hopefully cause a return of spontaneous circulation (ROSC).

5. **(T)** F Dopamine is indicated for treating hypotension secondary to congestive heart failure, myocardial infarction, trauma, sepsis, and overt heart failure.

6. T **(F)** Dopamine is administered via intramuscular injection.

7. T **F** A patient's cardiovascular history has no effect on the administration of ROCM.

8. **T** F Extravasation of IV sodium bicarbonate can lead to tissue necrosis.

Multiple-Choice Questions

Place a check before the letter of the correct answer.

1. The highest survival rate following cardiac arrest occurs in patients who receive CPR within what time frame?
   _____ **a.** 4 minutes
   _____ **b.** 6 minutes
   _____ **c.** 8 minutes
   _____ **d.** 10 minutes

2. Epinephrine is the pharmaceutical equivalent to which of the following?
   _____ **a.** Renin
   _____ **b.** Adrenaline
   _____ **c.** Aldosterone
   _____ **d.** ADH

3. The antidiuretic hormone known as which of the following is a potent vasoconstrictor?
   _____ **a.** Adrenaline
   _____ **b.** Xylocaine
   _____ **c.** Nitroglycerin
   _____ **d.** Vasopressin

4. What is the term for a drug that inhibits the postganglionic parasympathetic receptors?
   _____ **a.** Antimuscarinic
   _____ **b.** Cholinergic
   _____ **c.** Sympathetic
   _____ **d.** Antidysrhythmic
   _____ **e.** Both a and b

5. What is the drug of choice when a patient exhibits bradycardia on the cardiac monitor?
   _____ **a.** Dopamine
   _____ **b.** Epinephrine
   _____ **c.** Atropine
   _____ **d.** Sodium bicarbonate
   _____ **e.** None of the above

6. Which of the following is a strong alkalinizing agent prescribed following cardiac arrest?
   _____ **a.** Epinephrine
   _____ **b.** Sodium bicarbonate
   _____ **c.** Atropine
   _____ **d.** Calcium

7. Dopamine should be delivered only via which of the following?
   _____ **a.** Intramuscular injection
   _____ **b.** Intraosseous injection
   _____ **c.** Intravenous injection
   _____ **d.** Endotracheal injection

8. Which drug is prescribed to convert a premature ventricular contraction to normal sinus rhythm?
   _____ **a.** Lidocaine
   _____ **b.** Sodium bicarbonate
   _____ **c.** Atropine
   _____ **d.** Epinephrine

Review Questions

1. In detail, what are the steps to be taken when an intravenous pyelogram patient suffers a cardiac arrest?

   1 - Call 4 Help   2 - State Location   8 - become familia
   3 - repeat it 3 times   4 - Start CPR   w/ meds
   5 - give correct meds ahead of time   9 - location of box
   6 - replace outdated meds   7 - stock room   10 - use of meds

2. What are the pharmacodynamic effects of alpha versus beta receptors?

   Alpha 1 = ↑ BF, dialates pupils, ↓ urination + pheces op
   Alpha 2 = ↓ BF, causes constipation
   Beta 1 = ↑ HR, ↑ CO, causes fat to break down,
   releases renin from kidneys
   Beta 2 = ↓ BP, opens airways, causes constipation,
   ↓ urine op, ↑ glucose productions, releases
   insulin, contracts skeletal muscle.

Answer Section

CHAPTER 1

Abbreviations

1. JRCERT: Joint Review Committee on Education in Radiologic Technology
2. ASRT: American Society of Radiologic Technologists

True-False

1. F
2. T
3. T
4. F
5. T
6. F
7. T
8. F
9. F
10. F

Discussion Questions

1. Because of the ever-changing legislative statutes within states, it is beyond the scope of this textbook to list current laws. Contact your state professional society regarding the most current restrictions.
2. Again, standards of care vary from state to state and even vary within states. Check with your professional society to verify the standard of care in your region concerning administration of pharmaceuticals.
3. The hospital and department policy manuals should outline in detail your responsibilities and limitations during a patient crisis. If they do not, all parties involved in resolving the crisis may be open to litigation.
4. There is no "correct" answer here. Discuss the situation with your fellow students and professor. What will your clinical facility allow you to do?
5. Begin with your state professional organization. Quickly involve state legislators elected from your district.
6. Negligence is the failure to do something that a reasonable person of ordinary prudence would do in a certain situation. Malpractice is a breach of duty to adhere to a standard of care.
7. Check your departmental policy manual.
8. Make sure that you are covered—in writing.
9. Yes or no? If they do continue to administer drugs, do they truly understand the ramifications?
10. Discuss the different answers with your fellow students.

CHAPTER 2

Abbreviations

1. AHA: American Hospital Association
2. AHFS: American Hospital Formulary Service
3. BNDD: Bureau of Narcotics and Dangerous Drugs
4. DEA: Drug Enforcement Agency
5. FDA: Food and Drug Administration
6. PDR: *Physician's Desk Reference*
7. POMR: Problem-oriented medical record

True-False

1. T
2. F
3. F
4. T
5. F
6. T
7. F
8. T
9. F
10. T
11. T

Review Questions

1. Controlled substance
2. Greater
3. Animal studies and human studies
4. *PDR, Facts and Comparisons, AHFS Drug Information, Mosby's GenRx, Handbook on Injectable Drugs, Drug Interaction Facts, Hansten's Drug Interactions, Drugs in Pregnancy and Lactation*
5. Medication name, date, dosage, route, and time; technologist's initials should also be recorded.
6. Patient's name, date order is written, medication name, dosage, route, frequency of dosage, and prescriber's signature.

Multiple-Choice Questions

1. c
2. b
3. d
4. a
5. d
6. b

CHAPTER 3

Review Questions

1. Fastest: solutions; slowest: enteric-coated tablets
2. Cardiac output, regional blood flow, drug reservoirs
3. Kidneys, intestines, respiratory system
4. An affinity for fat

5. They are: (1) the nature of the absorbing surface through which the drug must go; (2) blood flow to the site of administration; (3) solubility of the drug; (4) pH; (5) drug concentration; and (6) dosage form.

6. Passive diffusion is the random movement of a substance from a region of higher concentration to a region of lower concentration until equilibrium is established at the membrane. The majority of drugs are transported via this mechanism. Active transport is conducted by "carriers" that form complexes with drug molecules on one surface of the membrane, carry them through the membrane, and then let them go. The ionic forms of most drugs do not readily enter cells and therefore require active transport. Active transport is usually more rapid than passive diffusion.

Fill-in-the-Blank Questions

1. The blood-brain barrier and the placental barrier are two drug distribution barriers the body has that are made of biologic membranes.
2. Biotransformation is another name for metabolism.
3. Biopharmaceutics is the area of pharmacology that focuses on the method for achieving effective drug administration.
4. Pharmacokinetics includes the processes of how a drug is absorbed, metabolized, distributed, and eliminated throughout the body.
5. The most common way drugs traverse cellular membranes is passive diffusion.
6. Active transport can move a drug from an area of low concentration to an area of higher concentration.
7. Medications must go through disintegration and dissolution in order to be absorbed across a cell membrane.

Matching

1. f	5. b
2. c	6. g
3. a	7. d
4. e	8. h

Multiple-Choice Questions

1. d	5. c
2. d	6. d
3. b	7. b
4. c	8. a

CHAPTER 4

True-False

1. F	6. F
2. F	7. T
3. T	8. F
4. F	9. F
5. T	10. T

Fill-in-the-Blank Questions

1. Generally thought to be catalysts responsible for changes in biochemical reactions, enzymes occur throughout the body systems.
2. A side effect is a predictable pharmacologic action on body systems other than those intended.
3. When two drugs are combined and cause a pharmacologic response that is greater than it would have been if the drugs had been given individually, this is known as synergism.
4. The method by which a drug elicits effects is known as the mechanism of action.
5. The organ is which the desired effect occurs is generally called the target organ.
6. A drug-enzyme interaction occurs when a drug resembles the substrate to which an enzyme usually attaches.
7. After drug administration the amount that reaches and remains in the systemic circulation depends on the rate and extent of absorption, distribution, metabolism, and elimination.
8. Any unwanted effect from a drug is termed adverse.
9. Both toxic and allergic effects are known as adverse.
10. A drug-drug interaction occurs when two or more drugs act in unison to produce additive agonist, synergistic, or antagonist responses.

Multiple-Choice Questions

1. b	5. d
2. c	6. d
3. c	7. b
4. b	8. d

Review Questions

1. Dosage was well above that required for peak drug performance.
2. Drug-receptor interactions, drug-enzyme interactions, and nonspecific drug interactions.
3. When two or more drugs act in unison; produces additive agonist, synergistic, or antagonist responses.

4. The higher the dose, the greater the toxic effects; dose may become toxic if metabolism or elimination is impaired.

CHAPTER 5
Abbreviations

ROCM: radiopaque contrast media

True-False Questions

1. F	**5.** T
2. T	**6.** F
3. F	**7.** T
4. T	

Multiple-Choice Questions

1. b	**5.** a
2. d	**6.** d
3. c	**7.** b
4. b	

Fill-in-the-Blank Questions

1. A <u>negatively</u> charged particle is known as an anion, and a <u>positively</u> charged particle is known as a cation.
2. A <u>highly osmotic agent</u> will attract water so that a dilutional effect can occur to equalize pressures between two permeable or semipermeable membranes.
3. <u>Increased</u> density of the ROCM alters the attenuation of x-rays, thus enhancing the anatomic image on the radiographic film.
4. <u>Iodine</u> is an integral component in ROCM because radiopacity is produced by this element.
5. <u>Intravascular</u> ROCM are excreted primarily via the kidneys and are concentrated in the kidneys.
6. <u>Intravascular</u> ROCM consist of large molecules, with molecular weights ranging from 600 to 1700 and with poor lipid solubility.

Review Questions

1. Ratio of iodine atoms to osmotically active particles is 3:2 in ratio-1.5 media and 3:1 in ratio-3.0 media.
2. Because it absorbs x-ray photons, thus enhancing contrast.
3. Large molecules that cannot cross cell membranes.
4. Excreted by the hepatobiliary system.
5. High-osmolality ionic ROCM, low-osmolality nonionic ROCM, and low-osmolality ionic ROCM.
6. When barium sulfate suspension is potentially harmful, such as in GI perforation, or when computed tomography is being used because of less artifact production.

CHAPTER 6
Abbreviations

1. DSA: digital subtraction angiography
2. EMD: electromechanical dissociation
3. ARF: acute renal failure

True-False Questions

1. F	**6.** T
2. T	**7.** T
3. F	**8.** F
4. T	**9.** T
5. F	**10.** T

Multiple-Choice Questions

1. c	**6.** a
2. a	**7.** b
3. c	**8.** b
4. b	**9.** d
5. d	**10.** d

anaphal

Fill-in-the-Blank Questions

1. An immediately life-threatening systemic hypersensitivity reaction is known as <u>anaphylaxis.</u> (Anaphylactoid reaction or anaphylactic reaction is also correct.)
2. A <u>chemoreceptor</u> is a sensory nerve cell activated by chemical stimuli.
3. ROCM can lead to sickling of red blood cells as a result of osmotic fluid shifts in patients who suffer from <u>sickle cell anemia.</u>
4. ROCM cross <u>placental barriers</u> and should not be used in pregnant women unless benefits far exceed risks.
5. Patients at risk for <u>ARF</u> following intravascular ROCM include those with preexisting renal compromise, diabetes with concomitant renal dysfunction, or dehydration.
6. Signs and symptoms of <u>thyroid storm</u> include fever, tachycardia, diaphoresis, agitation, nervousness, and emotional instability.
7. Because of the serious effects that can occur by injection of intravascular ROCM, the imaging technologist should use a screening method that includes <u>the assessment of patient medical history</u> and <u>current renal function status.</u>
8. <u>Vasodilators</u> are used to improve delivery of ROCM to small arteries that may be inaccessible otherwise.

Review Question

1. Mast cells may respond to the first exposure with anaphylaxis.
2. Assume incompatibility and flush line with saline to prevent drug-drug contact.

CHAPTER 7
Abbreviations

1. SC: subcutaneous
2. IM: intramuscular
3. IV: intravenous

True-False

1. F
2. T
3. F
4. F
5. T
6. T
7. T
8. F

Multiple-Choice Questions

1. a
2. c
3. b
4. b
5. b
6. d
7. b
8. c
9. b
10. b

Review Questions

1. They are: (1) injection site should at a considerable distance from large nerves, bones, and blood vessels and from bruised, scarred, or swollen previous injection sites; (2) the proper needle length and gauge should be selected based upon injection site, tissue condition, size of patient, and the type of drug to be injected; (3) hold needle and syringe assembly as if it were a dart, and make the injection perpendicular to the skin surface from a distance of about 2 inches, in one quick motion; (4) aspirate to determine proper needle location (not in a blood vessel); (5) inject medication; (6) massage site to disperse the drug.

2. Ask patient to lie face down to expose the dorsogluteal site for identification of landmarks (greater trochanter of the femur to the posterior iliac spine) for injection anywhere along this imaginary line; or ask patient to lie on either side to locate landmarks on the left side, the technologist should palpate for the left greater trochanter with the right palm, point the right index finger to the anterior superior iliac spine, and extend the middle finger toward the iliac crest—and inject into the center of the V formed between the index finger and the middle finger (use left hand to detect landmarks in the right hip).

CHAPTER 8
Abbreviations

1. CDC: Centers for Disease Control and Prevention
2. BSP: body substance precautions
3. IDU: intravenous drug user
4. HBV: hepatitis B virus
5. OSHA: Occupational Safety and Health Administration

True-False

1. T
2. F
3. T
4. T
5. F
6. F
7. F
8. T

Multiple-Choice Questions

1. c
2. d
3. b
4. d
5. c
6. d
7. b
8. a
9. a

Review Questions

1. During recapping, it is very easy to be distracted or slip and puncture your finger or hand with the contaminated needle. Simply throw the entire needle and syringe away in a clearly marked "sharps" disposal box.

2. They are: (1) gloves should be worn when in contact with blood, body fluids containing visible blood, mucous membranes, or nonintact skin; (2) gloves should be worn when handling items or touching surfaces soiled with blood or body fluids and when performing venipuncture and other vascular access procedures; (3) gloves should be changed after contact with each patient; (4) masks and protective eye shields should be worn during procedures that can generate droplets of blood or other body fluids, to prevent exposure of mucous membranes of the mouth, nose, and eyes to infections; (5) gowns should be worn during procedures that can result in the splashing of blood or other body fluids; (6) hands and other skin surfaces should be thoroughly washed immediately after contamination with blood or body fluids; (7) needles should not be recapped, purposely bent or broken, or removed from syringes; (8) needles and syringes must be disposed of in puncture-resistant containers in the immediate work area; (9) mouthpieces, ambu bags, and ventilation devices should be used rather than mouth-to-mouth resuscitation; (10) health care workers with oozing or open sores should refrain from direct contact and handling of patient care equipment or items.

CHAPTER 9
True-False

1. T
2. F
3. F
4. T
5. T
6. F
7. T

Fill-in-the-Blank Questions

1. Extravasation is the accidental injection of IV fluid or medication into the tissues surrounding the vein.
2. The area in front of the elbow (the bend) is known as antecubital space.
3. A(n) hematoma is a collection of blood in the tissues of the skin or an organ.
4. A(n) intermittent-injection port (sometimes called a heparin lock) is a small adapter with a diaphragm that is attached to an IV catheter when more than one injection is anticipated.
5. Checking for backflow, immobilizing the needle at the injection site, and stopping the injection immediately if the patient complains of discomfort are three ways to minimize the possibility of extravasation.
6. Obese patients may have veins that are too deep to be seen or palpated; elderly patients may have veins that are easily seen but that may roll under the skin.
7. The two most common replacement fluids for dehydrated patients are normal saline and a 5% solution of dextrose in water.

Review Questions

1. Secure the tourniquet around the arm above the elbow; the ideal vein can be readily seen and palpated and should be at least twice the diameter of the needle or catheter used; if a suitable vein is still not apparent, hang the arm down for a few seconds, and then gently slap the skin over the site.
2. Remove the needle immediately; reassure the patient that the pain is temporary; maintain pressure on the vein until the bleeding has stopped; apply hot packs to the site to lessen pain.
3. Intravenously
4. Do not recap needles. Dispose of needles and syringes in a well-marked and safe "sharps" container.
5. Time of administration; drug name; dosage; route of administration; name of person delivering medication

CHAPTER 10
Abbreviations

1. ACLS: advanced cardiac life support
2. ADH: antidiuretic hormone
3. BLS: basic life support
4. AHA: American Heart Association
5. CPR: cardiopulmonary resuscitation

True-False

1. T
2. T
3. F
4. T
5. T
6. F
7. F
8. T

Multiple-Choice Questions

1. a
2. b
3. d
4. e
5. c
6. b
7. c
8. a

Review Questions

1. Call for help. Become familiar with the emergency paging system of the institution so that a swift summons for help can be done. State the location where help is needed. Repeat the summons at least three times before hanging up the paging system. Immediately after hanging up the paging system, initiate basic life support (BLS) by using proper cardiopulmonary resuscitation. In addition, the technologist should prepare in advance by checking the emergency medication box (or cart) to be certain that all medications and supplies are fresh. This is recommended to be done at least once every month. Replace any outdated medications or supplies. Make certain that there are adequate quantities of medications and supplies, restocking if necessary. Finally, become familiar with the pharmacology of emergency drugs, their locations within the box, and their proper use.
2. $alpha_1$: increases blood pressure, dilates pupils, decreases ability to urinate and defecate
   $alpha_2$: decreases blood pressure (when stimulated in the brain), causes constipation
   $beta_1$: increases heart rate, cardiac output, and dysrhythmias; causes fat to break down (lipolysis); releases renin hormone from the kidneys (may lead to increased blood pressure)
   $beta_2$: decreases blood pressure, opens airways, causes constipation, inhibits uterine contractions, increases glucose production, releases insulin, contracts skeletal muscle
   The above effects are seen when the receptor is stimulated; if more than one receptor is stimulated at any given moment, the effects seen may be mixed.

Bibliography

American Hospital Association Guide to the Health Care Field, Chicago, 1994, American Medical Association.

American Registry of Radiologic Technologists Educator's Handbook, ed 3, Mendota Heights, Minn, 1990, AART.

American Society of Health-Systems Pharmacists: *AHFS Drug Information 1995,* Bethesda, Md, 1995, The Society, pp 1671-1722.

American Society of Radiologic Technologists: Majority representation, *ASRT Scanner,* vol 23, no 4, April-May 1991.

Amin MM, Chan RH, Dunnick RN: Ionic and nonionic contrast media: current status and controversies, *Appl Radiol,* November 1993, pp 41-53.

Apker C: Appropriate application of contrast media: ionic vs nonionic, *Decisions in Imaging Economics,* 4:52-56, 1995.

Baker ME, Beam C, Leader R, et al: Contrast material for combined abdominal and pelvis CT: can cost be reduced by increasing the concentration and decreasing the volume? *Am J Roentgenol* 160:637-640, 1993.

Bernardino ME, Fishman EK, Jeffrey RB Jr, Brown PC: Comparison of Iohexol 300 and Diatrizoate Meglumine 60 for body CT: image quality, adverse reactions and aborted/repeated examinations, *Am J Roentgenol* 158:665-667, 1992.

Bettmann MA, Morris TW: Recent Advances in Contrast Agents, *Radiol Clin North Am* 24(3):347-357, 1986.

Brody TM, Larner J, Minneman KP, Neu HC: *Human pharmacology: molecular to clinical,* ed. 2, St Louis, 1995, Mosby.

Dawson P: Embolic problems in angiography, *Semin Hematol* 28(4)(suppl 7):31-37, 1991.

Dawson P, Strickland NH: Thromboembolic phenomena in clinical angiography: role of materials and technique, *JVIR* 2:125-132, 1991.

Dunnick RN, Cohan RH: Cost, corticosteroids and contrast media (commentary), *Am J Roentgenol* 162:527-529, 1994.

Edmunds MW: Preparing and administering medications. In *Introduction to clinical pharmacology,* ed 2, St Louis, 1995, Mosby, pp 41-91.

Ehrlich RA, McCloskey ED: *Patient care in radiography,* ed 4, St Louis, 1993, Mosby.

Evens RG: Economic impact of low-osmolarity contrast agents on radiology procedure and departments, *Radiology* 162:267-268, 1987.

Gavant ML, Ellis JV, Kleges LM: Diagnostic efficacy of excretory urography with low-dose nonionic contrast media, *Radiology* 182:657-660, 1992.

Hatfield S: Venipuncture makes way into radiologic science curricula, *Adv Radiol Sci Prof,* January 13, 1992, p 5.

Hilal S: Hemodynamic changes associated with intra-arterial injection of contrast media, *Radiology* 86:615-633, 1966.

Hill JA, Grabowski EF: Relationship of anticoagulation and radiographic contrast agents to thrombosis during coronary angiography and angioplasty: are there real concerns? *Cathet Cardiovasc Diagn* 25:200-208, 1992.

Hopper KD, Lambe H, Matthews YL: Current usage of nonionic contrast, *Urol Radiol* 14:218-220, 1992.

Hou SH, Bushinsky DA, Wish JB, et al: Hospital-acquired renal insufficiency: a prospective study, *Am J Med* 141:1027-1033, 1983.

Irving HD, Burbridge BE: Incompatibility of contrast agents with intravascular medications, *Radiology* 173:91-92, 1989.

Jacobson PD, Rosenquist CJ: *The diffusion of low osmolarity contrast agents: technological change and defensive medicine,* Santa Monica, Calif, 1994, Rand Corp.

Katayama H, Yamaguchi K, Kozuka T, et al: Adverse reactions to ionic and nonionic contrast media: a report from the Japanese Committee on the Safety of Contrast Media, *Radiology* 175:621-628, 1990.

Keefer BS: Facing the risk, *RT Image* 5:32, August 10, 1992.

Kelly J: A drug problem, *RT Image* 7:36, September 5, 1994.

Kim SH, Lee HK, Han MC: Incompatibility of water-soluble contrast media and intravascular pharmacologic agents: an in vitro study, *Invest Radiol* 27:45-49, 1992.

Kowalczyk N, Donnett K: *Integrated patient care for the imaging professional,* St Louis, 1996, Mosby.

Lasser EC, Berry CC, Mishkin MM, et al: Pretreatment with corticosteroids to prevent adverse reactions to nonionic contrast media, *Am J Roentgenol* 162:523-526, 1994.

Laurie AJ, Lyon SG, Lasser EC: The effects of contrast media on coagulation factor XII, *Invest Radiol* 26:S23-S25, 1991.

Levin DC, Gardiner GA, Karasick S, et al: Cost containment in the use of low-osmolar contrast agents: effect of guidelines monitoring and feedback mechanisms, *Radiology* 189:753-757, 1993.

Loudin A: Preparing for venipuncture, *RT Image,* 4(24):1, June 17, 1991.

Manual on Iodinated Contrast Media, Reston, Va, 1991, American College of Radiology.

McClennan BL: Ionic and nonionic iodinated contrast media: evaluation and strategies for use, *Am J Roentgenol* 155:225-233, 1990.

McKenry LM, Salerno E: Principles of drug action. In *Mosby's Pharmacology in Nursing,* ed. 20, St Louis, 1998, pp 29-48.

McTernan EJ, Hawkins RO: *Educating personnel for the allied health professions and services,* St Louis, 1972, Mosby.

Mishkin MM: Use of iodinated contrast agents: principles and practice, *Decisions in Imaging Economics* 4:15-17, 1991.

Mixdorf M, Goldsworthy R: The radiography essentials: an evolutionary perspective, *Radiol Technol* 63:386, 1992.

Morris TW, Fischer H: The pharmacology of intravenous radiocontrast media, *Ann Rev Pharmacol Toxicol* 26:143-160, 1986.

Morris TW, Francis M, Fischer HW: A comparison of the cardiovascular responses to carotid injections of ionic and nonionic contrast media, *Invest Radiol* 14(3):217-223, 1979.

Peppers MP: Pharmacologic mechanisms of radiologic contrast media, *Semin Radiol Technol* 3(3):163-171, 1995.

Peppers MP: Pharmacologic poisoning. In *Principles and practice of intensive care medicine,* Philadelphia, 1993, WB Saunders Co, pp 1702-1714.

Peppers MP: Understanding pharmacology, *Emergency* 25(1):18-26, 1993.

Pila TJ, Beshany SE, Shields JB: Incompatibility of Hexabrix and papaverine, *Am J Roentgenol* 146:1300-1301, 1986.

Poteet M: Venipuncture: has the time come? *Wavelength* 3(1):1, October 1991.

Reasner CA, Isley WL: Thyrotoxicosis in the critically ill, *Crit Care Clin* 7(1):57-74, 1991.

Roberts GH, Carson J: Venipuncture tips for radiologic technologists, *Radiol Technol* 65(2):107-112, 1993.

Rutledge DR, Geheb MA, Cronin S, Peppers MP: Pharmacokinetics in critically ill patients. In *Principles and practice of intensive care medicine,* Philadelphia, 1993, WB Saunders Co, pp 1686-1701.

Sage MR: Kinetics of water soluble contrast media in the central nervous system, *Am J Roentgenol* 141:815-824, 1983.

Shealey BA: Injecting pharmaceuticals: does hospital staff know the facts? *Adv Radiol Sci Prof* 9:3, February 5, 1996.

Spataro RF: New and old contrast agents: pharmacology, tissue opacification, and excretory urography, *Urol Radiol* 10:2-5, 1988.

Standards for an Accredited Educational Program in Radiologic Sciences, Chicago, 1997, Joint Review Committee on Education in Radiologic Technology.

Swanson DP, Jurgens RW: Radiopaque contrast media: the role of the pharmacist, *J Pharm Pract* 2(3):162-170, 1989.

Tortorici MR: *Task analysis of special procedures radiography and computerized axial tomography technology,* dissertation, Houston, 1979, University of Houston.

Tortorici MR, MacDonald JM: RTs performing venipuncture: a survey of state regulations, *Radiol Technol* 64(6):368, 1993.

Zeich J: Can we afford to use nonionic contrast? *Diagn Imaging Clin Med,* April 1989, pp 67-73.

Index

Illustration Credits

NOTES

NOTES

NOTES

NOTES

NOTES

NOTES

NOTES

NOTES

NOTES